Paediatric
Clinical
Examination
Made Easy

KU-529-552

BRITISH MEDICAL ASSOCIATION

1002015

To our children: Kieron, Daniel, Aisling, Meagan, Michael, Slaney, Eoin, Cliona, Helene and Aisling and to our respective wives, Margaret and Helene

For Elsevier:
Content Strategist: Pauline Graham
Content Development Specialist: Humayra Rahman Khan
Project Manager: Andrew Riley
Designer: Margaret Reid
Marketing Manager: Deborah Watkins

Paediatric Clinical Examination Made Easy

Denis Gill MB BSc DCH FRCPI FRCPCH
Professor of Paediatrics, Royal College of Surgeons in
Ireland and The Children's University Hospital, Dublin,
Ireland

Niall O'Brien MB DCH FRCPI
Consultant Paediatrician, National Maternity Hospital and
The Children's University Hospital, Dublin, Ireland

Illustrated by Des Hickey

SIXTH EDITION

BMA LIBRARY
WITHDRAWN
FROM LIBRARY
BRITISH MEDICAL ASSOCIATION

ELSEVIER

Search full text online at StudentConsult.Com
EDINBURGH LONDON NEW YORK PHILADELPHIA ST LOUIS
SYDNEY TORONTO 2018

ELSEVIER

© Longman Group UK Limited 1993
© Pearson Professional Limited 1996
© Harcourt Health Sciences Limited 1998
© Elsevier Science Limited 2002
© 2007 Elsevier Limited. All rights reserved
© 2018 Elsevier Limited. All rights reserved

The right of Denis Gill and Niall O'Brien to be identified as authors of this work has been asserted by them in accordance with the Copyright, Designs and Patents Act 1988.

No part of this publication may be reproduced, stored in a retrieval system, or transmitted in any form or by any means, electronic, mechanical, photocopying, recording or otherwise, without the prior permission of the Publishers. Permissions may be sought directly from Elsevier's Health Sciences Rights Department, 1600 John F. Kennedy Boulevard, Suite 1800, Philadelphia, PA 19103-2899, USA: phone: (+1) 215 239 3804; fax: (+1) 215 239 3805; or, e-mail: healthpermissions@elsevier.com. You may also complete your request on-line via the Elsevier homepage (http://www.elsevier.com), by selecting 'Support and contact' and then 'Copyright and Permission'.

First edition 1993
Second edition 1996
Third edition 1998
Fourth edition 2002
Fifth edition 2007
Sixth edition 2018

ISBN: 978-0-7020-7288-8
International Edition ISBN: 978-0-7020-7289-5

Note
Neither the Publisher nor the Authors assume any responsibility for any loss or injury and/or damage to persons or property arising out of or related to any use of the material contained in this book. It is the responsibility of the treating practitioner, relying on independent expertise and knowledge of the patient, to determine the best treatment and method of application for the patient.

ELSEVIER your source for books, journals and multimedia in the health sciences

www.elsevierhealth.com

Working together to grow libraries in developing countries

www.elsevier.com | www.bookaid.org | www.sabre.org

ELSEVIER   BOOK AID International   Sabre Foundation

The publisher's policy is to use **paper manufactured from sustainable forests**

Printed in China

Preface to Sixth Edition

One of the pleasures of writing the preface for a book on clinical examination is that the fundamentals don't change. A thorough history, a complete physical examination and a logical deduction and conclusion from the findings remain the basis of clinical interaction. In this edition, we have responded to critiques by adding extra diagrams, making alterations here and there, and improving the layout. The good doctor is the good listener, good examiner, good interpreter and good problem-solver. We hope that clinical examination will not be supplanted by CTs, MRIs, PETs, and increasingly sophisticated scanning techniques. Scanning techniques have improved dramatically in the past 20 years for those based in secondary and tertiary care hospitals. This has been especially true of ultrasonic examinations of the acute abdomen in infants and children, in cardiac echographs, and in MRI examination of the newborn and infant brain, to cite but a few examples. The primary care paediatrician working in remote or isolated practice will still need to rely on his/her diagnostic wit and clinical skills. We trust that clinical findings will continue to direct appropriate investigations. Listening and laying on of hands remain the cornerstones of clinical contact and contract. Good children's clinicians do more talking and thinking, and hopefully less blood testing. Children will like them for that.

Denis Gill
Niall O'Brien

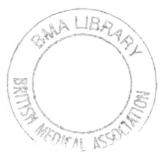

BMA LIBRARY BRITISH MEDICAL ASSOCIATION

Acknowledgements

We could not have delivered the text without the tireless typing of Norma McEneaney, the photographic shots of Thomas Nolan, and the lively illustrations of Des Hickey; to all of them we are extremely grateful. We thank Professor Alan Browne for his view of the Hippocratic tradition.

D.G.G.
N.O'B

Internet sites

There is virtually limitless information available on the internet. Students will learn of and access their favourite sites. The list below is limited and selective, but hopefully contains appropriate starting points.

- http://journals.bmj.com   *BMJ* (British Medical Journal)
- www.medicalstudent.com
- www.aap.org   American Academy of Pediatrics
- www.omim.org Online Mendelian Inheritance in Man
- http://www.medic8.com/MedicalDictionary.htm
- www.rarediseases.org
- http://www.ncbi.nim.nih.gov/pubmed   PubMed
- www.rcpch.ac.uk   Royal College of Paediatrics and Child Health
- www.cdc.gov   Centers for Disease Control and Prevention (CDC)
- http://www.who.int/en/   World Health Organization (WHO)
- http://adc.bmj.com/   *Archives of Disease in Childhood*
- http://student.bmj.com/student/student-bmj.html *Student BMJ*

Contents

1 Introduction

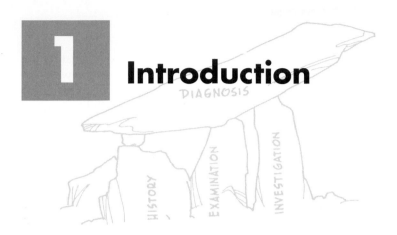

DIAGNOSIS

HISTORY   EXAMINATION   INVESTIGATION

The text is aimed at undergraduate medical students taking their paediatric course and also at postgraduate doctors commencing their first post in paediatrics. Experience has taught us that paediatric residents frequently need to refresh and retrain themselves in child health and disease. The term 'student' refers therefore to both postgraduate and undergraduate students of paediatrics. Strange though it may seem, undergraduate and postgraduate education are interrelated. The medical graduate has an inherent obligation to remain a student for life. Our aims are to emphasize the important art of history taking both from parents and child, to guide in the elicitation and interpretation of physical signs in children of varying ages, and to provide some sources of further information.

Doctors caring for little children need to develop their observational and instinctual skills. Occasionally the combination of an observational clue plus an instinctual cue can result in 'instant diagnosis'. Throughout we wish to emphasize the value of attentive observation.

Our approach is essentially clinical, and will be confined largely to symptoms and signs. This does *not* purport to be a textbook of paediatrics and no effort is made to include descriptions of syndrome identification, clinical conditions, laboratory investigations or treatment protocols. These can all be found in standard textbooks. Our objective is to expand the first few chapters of the basic text into a child-centred clinical approach towards problem solving in paediatrics.

We believe that the simple but subtle skills of physical examination and history taking are essential if one is to be a dedicated doctor to children. Too many students spend inappropriate time in the library at the expense of being at the bedside. Our philosophy is that the student cannot examine too many babies, infants or children. To know the abnormal, you must first know the normal.

We suspect that medical students may be exposed to a surfeit of unusual cases and conditions at the expense of more common and mundane problems. Remember that what is common is common, and that one must be versed in the usual to become good at the unusual.

We have elected to concentrate mainly on the newborn, infant and preschool child, for these are the ages of greatest change and most difficulty. The schoolchild is rational and reasonable, and can usually be examined as a 'mini-adult' in an organized fashion.

This text is written on the understanding that students taking paediatrics have had previous exposure to clinical methods. No effort is made, therefore, to define basic clinical terms such as, for example, crepitations, clubbing or chorea. Studded through the text are boxes containing special paediatric terminology with which the student may experience difficulty. Textbooks sometimes display disease in its most florid form. Insufficient emphasis may be placed on nuances of disease and degrees of disorder. Implicit in paediatrics is an ability to recognize subtle signs of sickness and to be able to say with some certainty that a baby is 'off' or an infant is 'ill'. Early recognition of problems facilitates early intervention and, hopefully, prevention of complications.

CHILDREN AND DOCTORS

Children are brought to doctors for a multitude of reasons: to reassure regarding normality; to receive immunizations; for developmental checks; for recognition of rashes; and so on. Insofar as medical students are concerned, the following are the most important reasons for consultation:

- for diagnosis of an acute illness (otitis, respiratory, infection, convulsions, appendicitis, etc.)
- for diagnosis and/or investigation of a chronic illness (failure to thrive, recurrent wheeze, protracted diarrhoea, for example)
- for delay in reaching developmental milestones
- for advice on immunization, nutrition, growth, normal variations
- for reassurance of normality
- for recognition and/or confirmation of a syndrome complex.

We trust that students will enjoy this primer and point out to us its deficits as well as their own problems. Paediatrics (doctoring of little people) should, above all, be pleasurable. Think of your children's experience as being in a 'learning hospital' rather than a 'teaching hospital'.

Listen to and learn from children. And mimic their main attribute, that of a constantly questioning nature. Ask 'Why?' over and over again.

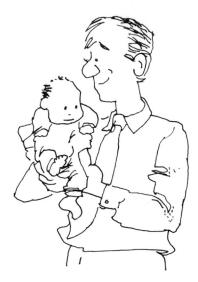

Fig. 1.1 Children are brought to doctors for a multitude of reasons.

- Look and you should see
- Ask and you should be answered.

The basic requirements needed to acquire the clinical skills in paediatrics are the same as those for adult medicine in the Hippocratic tradition.

Clinical skill	Requirement
history taking	education
physical examination	skill
diagnosis	inductive logic
prognosis	experience
treatment	knowledge

Sufficient incentive should be provided by the needs of children for good doctors, and by your need to pass your assessment. We do hope to transfer some of the skills required to examine children and to provide a flavour of the rewards to be obtained by good practice.

Recall at all times the ancient adage:

- I hear and forget
- I see and remember
- I do and understand.

'VETERINARY' PAEDIATRICS

By using the term 'veterinary' we are not attempting to be derogatory, but are trying to draw your attention to certain analogies between young children and animals. We also hope to persuade you to commence all examinations as veterinarians do – by listening and looking.

Some attributes shared by animals and small children are:

- they don't like being stared at
- they lie down when sick
- repeated food refusal is unusual
- they have limited ability to express themselves

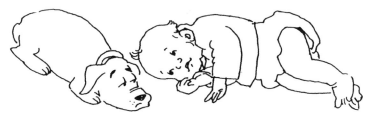

Fig. 1.2 'Veterinary paediatrics': small children and animals share certain characteristics.

- they adopt the position of comfort when well
- their survival instinct is strong.

Inspection and intuition are therefore important introductions to paediatric examination. Some cynic has coined the term 'paediatric zoology' to describe the collection and study of rare cases and conditions in teaching hospitals!

AIMS AND OBJECTIVES IN PAEDIATRICS

Every department of child health will set its own course aims and objectives. In broad terms they will include the following main headings:

1. To teach the recognition and management of the well and ill infant and child.
2. To emphasize the importance of growth and development of both the normal and the sick child.
3. To provide a sound basic knowledge of child health and disease.
4. To enable the student to acquire sufficient skill to carry out a full physical examination of a newborn infant, toddler, child and adolescent.
5. To demonstrate adequate medical, developmental, social and behavioural history taking from the parents or guardians of the child.
6. To stress the importance of the child's family and social background in relation to his well-being and illnesses.
7. To emphasize the importance of prevention in paediatrics; in particular, this applies to immunization, nutrition and avoidance of accidents.
8. To demonstrate the relationship between genetic and environmental factors in the causation of malformation and of illness.

9. To provide an understanding of the handicapping conditions of childhood and of the services available for their amelioration.

A student should set himself the more straightforward and simple targets:

1. To be able to elicit and interpret findings from history and physical examination.
2. To be able to construct a reasonable differential diagnosis and problem list.
3. To be able to prepare plans for appropriate investigation and management.
4. To be able to communicate adequately with children and with their parents.

THE SEVEN AGES OF CHILDREN

Children change, grow, mature and develop. One's style and approach to physical examination will very much depend on the child's age, independence and understanding. The seven ages of children are:

1. Newborn, neonate = first month of life
2. Infant = 1 month to 1 year
3. Toddler = 1 year to 3 years
4. Preschool child = 3–5 years
5. Schoolchild = 5–18 years
6. Child = 0–18 years
7. Adolescent = early: 10–14 years
   = late: 15–18 years.

Throughout the text the terms 'he', 'him', 'his', should be taken to be 'ambisextrous' and to refer to 'him' and 'her'. We reject the use of neuter 'it' in referring to children.

Paediatrics is the medical care of children up to the completion of growth and development.

CHILDREN IN HOSPITAL

It has been said that the primary function of paediatricians is to discharge children from hospital. In developed countries the average inpatient stay has dropped steadily and now has a mean of 2–4 days. Indeed many children only stay 1–2 days. Students need to be on their toes if they are to see and learn. About half of all admissions will be infants and toddlers – hence the importance, where possible, of an omnipresent parent.

Parallel with reduced inpatient stay has been an increased use of day care, both for medical and surgical purposes. Many of the most interesting and complicated paediatric cases are to be found having various procedures in the plastic, orthopaedic, urological and neurosurgical units.

Why are children in hospital?

- For care of acute and chronic illness
- For surgery, acute and elective
- For investigative, therapeutic and diagnostic procedures
- For multidisciplinary assessment, particularly if handicapped
- For their protection (in cases of serious non-accidental injury)
- For observation (in behavioural and other disorders)
- For social reasons.

In the future much of paediatrics will be practised on an 'ambulatory' basis – in the day ward, in the outpatient department and in the community clinic. During your paediatric course, visits to all these activities will be imperative. In addition, we recommend visits to child-oriented general practices, institutes for the mentally and physically handicapped, and vaccination sessions.

Inner-city children's hospitals tend to continue to have busy accident and emergency ('casualty') departments. In reality, a large proportion (as much as 50%) of the work of these departments relates to primary care problems: that is, medical conditions that should be handled in the community. We urge students to avail themselves of the opportunity to see the common problems in practice – respiratory infections, infectious illnesses, minor injuries, rashes, vague symptoms, etc., in the accident and emergency department. Remember that although leukaemia, nephrotic syndrome and epiglottitis may be relatively common conditions in hospital practice, they are distinctly rare in general practice. The general practitioner is more likely to encounter iron deficiency anaemia, urinary tract infection and viral 'croup' than any of the above.

By their nature, children's hospitals tend to have a disproportionate collection of curiosities and congenital disorders. Remember our rules:

1. First know the normal
2. Then know variants of normal
3. Then know abnormality, noting that: normality and abnormality are closely allied, and thin partitions do their bounds divide.

Some 5–7% of children are admitted to hospital annually, and some 50% of children have been in hospital by the age of 7 years. Observe the effects of hospitalization on children. Note the trauma of separation if a parent cannot be present. Learn of the efforts that are now being made to mitigate the effects of hospitalization on vulnerable children through preparation, play, parental accommodation, painting and, above all, pleasant hospital people, from porters to professors. Although nurses are nearly always nice and doctors do their best, students should be simple, straight and considerate in their approach to children. Remember the words

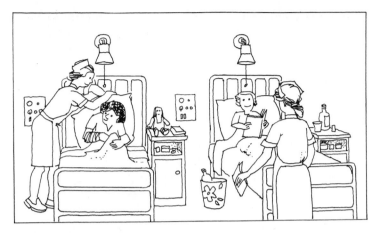

Fig. 1.3 Children on hospital ward.

of Marcus (aged 6) who wrote, 'Even nasty people are nice when you're ill'.

> When I was sick and lay a-bed
> I had two pillows at my head.
> And all my toys beside me lay
> To keep me happy all the day.
>
> Robert Louis Stevenson

THREE PILLARS OF DIAGNOSIS

Medical diagnosis rests on the traditional tripod of history, physical examination and investigation. Paediatric problem solving rests heavily on history, partly on examination (observation) and partly on investigation. A carefully taken and properly recorded history is the clinical keystone. The history should give prime emphasis to the mother's worries and reasons for bringing the child to the doctor. Physical

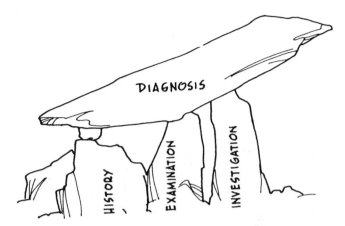

Fig. 1.4 The three pillars of diagnosis are history, physical examination and investigation.

examination, with its techniques, tricks and tribulations, is described in detail in other parts of this text. The results of examination need to be recorded in a standard legible style with due emphasis on relevant negative findings. The brief designation O/E NAD (on examination, nothing abnormal detected) is inadequate for undergraduate purposes.

With experience, a thorough examination of infants and children can be completed in a short time. Parents are very reassured by doctors who do a thorough examination, not merely confining themselves to the presenting part, be that a sore ear or a limp. There is simply no substitute for examining lots of normal children. Know the normal, and deviations can be subsequently recognized. Today's parents (of smaller families) want to know that their children are normal and, if not, what the matter is. Would you trust a doctor who failed to examine you, performed only a cursory inspection or examined only the apparent presenting problem?

- History is the keystone
- Examine the whole child
- See lots of children.

We shall not refer to investigation in this book, but rather refer you to your standard text.

> I seek a method by which the teachers teach less and learners learn more.
>
> Comenius (1630)

Clinical binary principles

two ears to listen
two eyes to look
two hands to examine
two hemispheres to deduce

> The skilful doctor knows what is wrong by observing alone, the middling doctor by listening, and the inferior doctor by feeling the pulse.
>
> Chang Chung-Ching (c150)

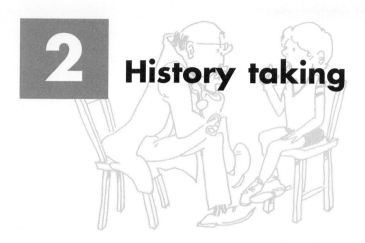

2 History taking

A smart mother makes often a better diagnosis than a poor doctor.

August Bier (1861–1949)

LISTENING TO MOTHERS

The most important attribute of any good doctor is to be a good listener. Listen carefully to mothers and note what they say. History is the vital cornerstone of paediatric problem solving. More important information is often gathered from a good history than from physical examination and laboratory investigation.

The first important ground rule in history taking is: *mother is right until proved otherwise*. Mothers are, by and large, excellent observers of their offspring and make good interpreters of their problems when sick. Even the most ill-educated mother will often surprise you by her intuition. She may not know what's wrong but she certainly knows something is wrong. If a mother says, 'I think my baby can't hear properly', the onus is on the doctor to corroborate or negate that statement.

In our view no one can replace the mother in providing an accurate and thorough description of the child and his complaints. Fathers will vary in their expertise, but often lack the information, insight and instinct that a good mother can provide. While the principle that mother is usually right prevails, the corollary must be that fathers can be off cue and off course. However, the modern day domesticated father is improving. Other caretakers – guardians, aunts, house-mothers – will vary widely in their knowledge of the child. We have been impressed by the inhibitory nature of some grandparents' presence at initial interviews and history taking.

At the outset it is important to try to establish a good rapport with the mother. Allow her to understand that you are more concerned with what she has to say than what Dr X has suggested. Make sure you understand her idiom and her concerns. A useful opening question is: 'What do you yourself think really is the cause of his trouble?' or 'Do you have any views as to what is wrong with him?'

These questions may lead you in the right direction. Alternatively, they may be important to negate following examination and investigation. Get into the habit of quoting verbatim from mother. Mothers frequently make statements whose importance, if not noted and recorded during history taking, may be subsequently lost. We both have the experience of saying to ourselves: 'If only I had listened to that mother; she was trying to tell me what was wrong'.

Students can unquestioningly accept a mother's complaints about her child without asking her to define her terms. Terms such as 'diarrhoea' or 'vomiting' require definition. Does diarrhoea mean frequent stools, semi-formed stools, offensive stools? Do you (or mother) know the normal frequency of stool passage? Is it reasonable to expect a teen-aged single parent to know children? What does the term 'hyperactivity' mean to you – are not all children active to varying degrees?

Listen to mother talking

- What are her worries?
- What does she think?
- Quote verbatim
- Understand her idiom
- Ask her to define her terms (What do you mean by . . . ?).

You need to establish that you are both talking about the same thing, be it croup, anorexia or breath-holding. You

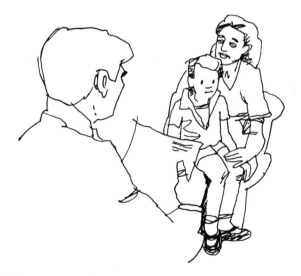

Fig. 2.1 Listen attentively to mother.

need also to learn her local idiom or slang (for example the penis may be referred to as the 'private parts', 'willy' or 'johnny'). In our hospital the residents have come to learn that when mothers say that the baby is 'lobbing and lying', they mean something serious is wrong. Australian mothers may state that the infant is 'crook'.

One needs to know the questions which produce the desired answers. A good opening ploy is, 'Tell me about your baby', and then simply let the mother talk. As you gain experience you will learn the important pointers and know when to interject succinct questions without interrupting her flow.

The student must of course take thorough notes interspersed with pithy quotations or spicy titbits. In time you'll learn how to cut corners, how to proceed down diagnostic avenues and how to recognize important cues. Learn through history taking (receiving) to be a good listener – to parents primarily, but also to your better teachers as they elicit clinical histories.

A poorly taken and recorded history

> Cough × 3 days
> Off feeds × 2 days
> Wheeze × 1 day
> Temperature × 1 day
> Vomit × 2.

Many current charts contain such anecdotal and unexplored facts. While the basic details are stated, there is inadequate inquisition and description. The diagnosis may then be recorded as 'chest infection', symptomatic of historical haziness and clinical laziness.

Always ask the parents to relate the sequence of events leading to the present complaints. A suitable start might be 'When was he last well? Which came first, the cough or the wheeze? In what way has he changed?' In eliciting the history of a convulsion, details of the time, place, surroundings, stimuli, etc., are of vital importance.

You will need also to obtain a general knowledge of the child. What sort of fellow is he? Is he active? Has he much energy? Is he outgoing, sociable? How does he sleep? Is school progress satisfactory? Is he developing normally? Whose side of the family does he resemble?

Let mothers talk

- Tell me about your baby
- What sort of fellow is he?
- When was he last well?
- Tell me what happened.

Patients also appreciate a doctor who gives them individ-ual attention and whose time is devoted to them (even though he may be in a hurry). Listen and you will hear. Time spent on history taking will be well repaid. Try to ensure that your written notes reflect adequately the time taken and interest shown. Some mothers do 'beat about the bush', dragging in all sorts of irrelevancies. With experience you will learn how to conduct and interrupt such garrulous gabblers.

Any of your standard texts and tutors will cite examples of how to fully explore a symptom, such as cough or pain.

When does it occur?
How long has he had it?
Can you describe it?
What brings it on?
Does anything relieve it?
How long does it last?
What is its pattern and periodicity?

Are there any associated symptoms?
What does he do when he has it?
What have you done about it?

This will necessarily be followed by a careful and thorough exploration of the relevant system, and then by a systems review. With time and experience, systems reviews tend to abbreviate and to become more precise. There is nothing special or different in paediatrics about the necessity of obtaining an adequate past history, family history and social history. Awareness of the child's place in the family, relationship with parents, siblings and peers, is crucial in obtaining a broad view of the child. So many of today's illnesses have social and behavioural overtones that the importance of the holistic view cannot be overemphasized.

A knowledge of the family's socioeconomic status, present financial situation, housing and employment is vital. Are the parents married, separated, cohabiting? Is the mother single? In some cases of handicap or metabolic disorder it will be prudent to enquire cautiously about consanguinity.

CUE WORDS

Computers accept key words; students ought to look out for *cue words* when taking histories. By cue words we mean simple statements, hidden in histories, which may be diagnostically alerting. Let us cite a few examples:

1. *Cue*: 'She does not like bread or biscuits.'
   Think: Could this be gluten enteropathy?
2. *Cue*: 'He just loves salt; he even licks it from things.'
   Question: Has he a salt losing state?
3. *Cue*: 'He's hungry after he vomits.'
   Answer: This is suggestive of mechanical vomiting, whether due to pyloric stenosis or gastro-oesophageal reflux.

4. *Cue*: 'He's always drinking, he'll drink anything, he'll even drink from toilet bowls.'
   Response: This sounds like true polydipsia.
5. *Cue*: 'I don't know where all the food goes.'
   Comment: When referred to a relatively inactive infant this statement may suggest a malabsorptive state, for example cystic fibrosis.

Mothers may, of course, unintentionally deceive. A common complaint is: 'I can't get him to eat anything.' And there in front of you sits a solemn, pudgy infant sucking on a bottle containing a mélange of milk, rusks, and maybe tea. In a similar vein, the seemingly contradictory statements, 'But he eats nothing doctor' followed rapidly by 'He never stops going' are frequently encountered. They usually reflect the overactive (and perhaps under-disciplined) toddler who is 'addicted to the bottle' and is consuming excessive carbohydrate by day and night.

A SAMPLE HISTORY

To obtain the right answers any detective must know how to ask (and frame) the right questions. This simple maxim applies to any system; nowhere is it more pertinent than in taking a history of a fit or convulsion. In any convulsion one needs to know as much as possible, about the child, his environment and the surrounding circumstances.

However, by way of example of a thorough history we have chosen the questioning of a mother whose child is wetting the bed (enuretic). This common complaint, source of much maternal irksomeness but often a dearth of medical interest, exemplifies the value of detailed and diligent history taking.

What age is he?
Where does he come in the family?
When did the bed wetting commence?

How frequently does he wet?
Does he wet by day?
How long can he retain his urine by day?
Does he have a good stream?
Has he had any kidney infections?
When was he dry by day?
Was dryness achieved easily or with difficulty?
Has he his own bed?
Does he awake when he wets?
Does he waken more than once per night?
Is he in nappies at night?
Who changes the sheets?
Have you inside toilets?
What have you done about wetting?
Does he want to be dry?
Has he had any dry nights?
What was his best dry period?
Is he dry when away?
Have you lifted him?
Have you restricted his fluids?
Have you reprimanded or punished him?
How does he get on at home and in school?
Have medication or alarms been tried?
Did any of his siblings wet at night?
Were either of you (his parents) wet when children?
How does the wetting affect him?
How does the wetting bother you?

This may seem like a ream of questions but with experience they can trip off the tongue promptly and buildup a picture of the child and his problem. Bed wetting is one of those complaints for which it can be useful to see the child and mother both together and separately.

Similar interrogation in depth can be constructed for a whole variety of symptoms from fits to fainting to feeding difficulties. There is simply no substitute for a thorough history, properly phrased and fully recorded, in diagnosing childhood disorders. Try writing one for asthma, abdominal pain or anaemia. Think of a suitable programme of questions one might feed into a computer and have the parents perform themselves while awaiting consultation.

Did you know that it has been estimated that about 70% of paediatric diagnoses are based mainly on *history*?

Summary 1

Eight-year-old boy. Recurrent chest infections particularly in winter. Nocturnal cough. Persistent runny nose. Past history of eczema. No physical findings today.
Impression: Asthma.

Summary 2

Two-year-old girl. Six-month history of diarrhoea. Stools are messy, loose and contain undigested food. Three to five bowel motions per day. Good energy, appetite. Normal height and weight for age. Well nourished. No findings.
Impression: Toddler diarrhoea ('peas and carrots syndrome').

Summary 3

Seven-year-old primary school girl. One-year history of staring, vacant episodes noted by parents and teacher. Eyes flicker. Child stops momentarily. Child not bothered by events. Carries on as if nothing has happened. Episodes occur two to three times per week. Occasionally two to three times per day. Normal intelligence, no past history, no physical findings.
Impression: Primary generalized epilepsy (absence seizures).

The above examples show that a good history with the pertinent points abstracted is the best pointer to diagnosis in paediatrics.

Help strategy

H = History
E = Examination
L = Logical deduction
P = Plan of management

Feeding history

Feeding is such an intrinsic part of infancy, and feeding problems so common, that a good history on feeding pattern and content is crucial. Too many doctors when presented with a feeding problem change the milk. The problem does not usually lie in the milk but in management of feeding and in the mother–infant relationship (harmonious or otherwise?). A detailed feeding history is vital if one is going to be able to discuss diet with today's allergy-conscious mothers.

Was the baby bottle or breast fed? If *breast fed*, what was the duration of exclusive breast feeding? Was this a satisfying experience for mother and baby? How often did she feed? Was he content? Were there any problems? How did he sleep, feed and gain? Did she feed on demand or to some sort of schedule? Was she complementing the breast milk with anything else?

If *bottle fed*, was he fed on formula or unmodified cow's milk? Which formula did he receive? How was it prepared? What volume did he take each feed and how long did he take over it? Frequency of feeds? Total daily intake? Any additives (iron or vitamins) given with milk? Duration of exclusive milk feeding?

Weaning

At what age were solids first introduced? Which solids? How were they administered – by spoon or in bottle? At what age were gluten-containing foods first given? Had he any preferences? When could he manage lumpy food?

Any known food allergies? Why do you think he is allergic to that substance? Does he suck well? Does he swallow well? What stops him feeding? Is it, for example, satiety, sleepiness or breathlessness? Were there weaning problems? How did you two get on? Did the father assist with bottle feeding? Do you feed him every time he cries? Do you give him drinks of water?

If all these questions fail to sort out the problem, one may have to resort to the request 'Show me how you do it please'.

Students can benefit from spending time doing nursing duties – changing, washing, holding and above all feeding babies. Learn by doing.

In conclusion, good history taking is the hallmark of the good student of paediatrics. In all histories it is imperative to get to the root of the problem. It may be worth repeating, now that you have established rapport with the parent, the following questions:

- Remind me again, why did you bring your child along?
- Just what are you worried about?
- What do you think is wrong with him?

A **full paediatric history** will enquire along the following general lines:

    pregnancy
    delivery

23

perinatal events
feeding practice
developmental progress
immunizations
infectious diseases
accidents and injuries
hospital admissions and operations
allergies
minor illnesses
medications
serial heights and weight, if known
school progress
travel.

During the taking of the history, preferably in relaxed surroundings, the opportunity should arise to observe how the child separates from the parent, how creatively and independently he plays, and occasionally how expressively he draws.

The whole history and nothing but the whole history

The full facts
The precise sequence of complaints
Changes noted since onset of illness

Insofar as students are concerned, the Ten Commandments of *record keeping* are:

Thou shalt write legibly
Thou shalt note the date and the time
Thou shalt record thorough histories and examinations
Thou shalt avoid abbreviations
Thou shalt write a succinct summary
Thou shalt list the important problems

Thou shalt make a diagnosis or, if not possible,
Thou shalt assemble a differential diagnosis
Thou shalt sign thy name and status
Thou shalt not alter entries.

LET THE CHILDREN SPEAK

While we repeatedly emphasize the value and importance of a mother's history of her child's complaints, don't forget the child. He may be very anxious to tell you his story and may have a useful contribution to make. Often, especially if he's verbally precocious and outgoing, or if he has a chronic condition and much experience of hospital, he may express himself remarkably lucidly. Children need to be heard and be seen to be noticed. They have a viewpoint which they are frequently eager to express. Children over 5 years should be asked to give their account of events with parental corroboration of certain points. One brief example. We recently saw

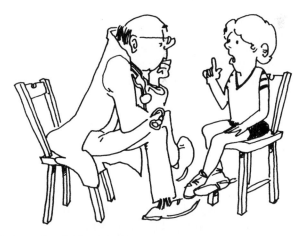

Fig. 2.2 Let the children speak!

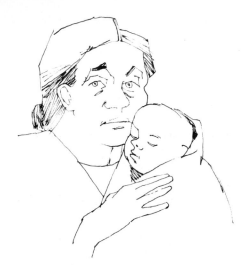

Fig. 2.3 An anxious mother with ill baby.

a bright 10-year-old boy with a proven duodenal ulcer. He described his pain as being 'like a laser beam going through my stomach'. Brilliant!

If he's reticent, shy or mute don't push him. He may talk later. Allowing him to draw himself, his family, their home may be revealing to those with psychological insight. Use of a tape recorder, or even a video (if your Department of Child Health is well equipped) can be useful, particularly in exploring behavioural or conduct problems.

Make sure you know the child's pet name as well as his given name. Laurence may be called 'Larry', Robert 'Bobby' and Catherine 'Katie'. In addition, the child recorded as Patrick Joseph, may in fact be called 'Junior'.

TALKING TO PARENTS

Parental anxiety is difficult to assess and can vary in degree from mild concern to severe emotional upset, sometimes culminating in aggressive behaviour. Being comfortable in discussions with parents comes from experience and observation of the approach used by more senior colleagues. Although there is no single correct approach, one must adapt to the great variation in paediatric conditions, from neonatal anomalies, through children with disabilities, to the otherwise healthy child with an acute illness. Preferably, both parents should be present, with the exclusion of other relatives unless parents insist.

In many cases both doctor and parents are strangers to each other. The initial approach will be a mutual assessment. A quick appraisal of the age of the parents, their education and social status may be helpful to the physician. It is important to show respect for the parents and, where possible, to avoid interruption during the discussion. Always use the child's name and be fully briefed in relation to age, previous history and if necessary sibling history. If appropriate, the child should be present and language and communication should reflect respect for the child concerned.

It is important to be as factual as can be whatever the circumstances, at the same time explaining the limitations of professional knowledge. When asked about statistical or percentage chances of recovery be careful to point out that each child is an individual. It is also pertinent in present times to have a witness from either medical or nursing staff present and to make a detailed note in the patient's chart.

Good listening is contributory to learning; good communication is the key to cooperative caring.

> **Parents of ill children broadly seek four degrees of information**
>
> 1. What is it? What is wrong?
> 2. What caused it? How did it happen?
> 3. What will be the outcome?
> 4. Will it happen again?

Clearly the answers to the above questions will considerably depend on whether the child's disorder is an acute one (e.g. meningitis) or whether it is an inherited abnormality (e.g. cleft palate). It is evident that one has difficulty responding to questions 2, 3 and 4 if one cannot answer question 1. Students should be reticent about discussing causes and consequences with parents until they possess the appropriate acumen and authority. Finally, don't forget the unvoiced (fifth) question:

Is it leukaemia, or cancer, or some lethal familial trait?

Could we, at the risk of sounding old fashioned and conservative, remind students to dress presentably. In your final years you are dealing with people as a trainee doctor rather than a science student. Many studies have shown that

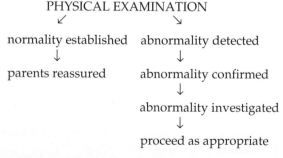

PHYSICAL EXAMINATION

↙   ↘

normality established   abnormality detected

↓   ↓

parents reassured   abnormality confirmed

↓

abnormality investigated

↓

proceed as appropriate

Fig. 2.4 Algorithm for action in consulting.

parents interact reluctantly with shabby, unshaven, scruffy students.

An initial office consultation perhaps should be the easiest to deal with. However, interpreting the history given – which may vary from one parent to another – can take time.

At some point you should ask the direct question, 'Is there some serious condition that you are worried or have read about?' The answer, in many cases, will get to the root of the problem, from where one can embark on physical assessment, appropriate investigations and possibly early management. (It is advisable to avoid meeting with relatives other than the parents, as in such circumstances the history may become more confusing.) In this day and age one must be prepared for extensive knowledge of some conditions acquired by parents from the internet, but remember that

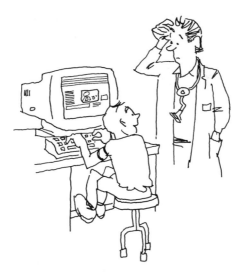

Fig. 2.5 In this day and age extensive knowledge can be acquired from the internet.

interpretation of such information is where the problem may lie.

BREAKING BAD NEWS TO PARENTS

As an undergraduate student, *don't*. You lack the authority, experience and acquired empathy. You can, however, learn the necessary attributes through communication skills exercises (videoed and later discussed), or better by sitting in on real scenarios in the hospital. Telling the parents that their newborn baby has Down's syndrome, or that their toddler has serious meningitis, or that the infant they rushed in for resuscitation has in fact died is always difficult, draining and demanding. The impact of bad news can be lessened if done quietly, sensitively and responsively.

- Speak slowly and simply
- Avoid medical terms
- Be as clear and concise as you can
- Don't try to transmit too much information
- Ask for questions
- Always have a nurse present
- Express your sympathy.

Never, never give bad news over the telephone. Give the news in private, appropriate surroundings. Allow parents time to express their shock, grief, guilt, anger, or whatever emotion.

Key paediatric points

Listen to mothers and note their concerns

Preverbal children's ability to communicate is limited. Learn to appreciate 'body language' and acquire some skills in observation (see p. 79)

Certain illnesses have predilections for certain ages:

bronchiolitis	<1 year
laryngotracheobronchitis	<3 years
transient synovitis	<5 years
slipped upper femoral epiphysis	~10 years.

As parents prepare to leave a discussion, always conclude by asking whether there are any points not clearly understood, or whether there are any further questions which they may have forgotten to ask.

3 Approaching children

Good current practice would suggest that all children of any age be examined by medical students only in the presence of a parent, guardian, nurse or chaperone. Examining children in the absence of a parent should only be carried out with their parent(s) consent and with the child's cooperation if old enough to give it.

THE APPROACH CODE

The first rules in approaching any child are very similar to those for crossing the road – stop, listen, look, then use your senses. The first approach is a hands-off one – *stop*. Allow the child to look at you and, insofar as he can, decide you are a person to be trusted. Let him look at you as you talk to his mother. Take your time, make no sudden moves (for you may frighten a fretful toddler) and be in no hurry to examine the child. Even better, let him play in your presence. Approach cautiously, be nice and utter reassuring sounds.

Listen to the mother. Children may come to the clinic, surgery or hospital in the company of a variety of caretakers (mother, father, guardian, foster-parent, nurse, relative). In our view, there is no substitute for the mother. She knows her child. The guiding principle in listening is: mother is usually right until or unless proved otherwise. We have expanded on this in Chapter 2. At the same time you may have the opportunity to listen to the child talk, relate to his mother, and to note his breathing, cough, stridor (if present) and other auditory phenomena such as his cry.

Then *look*. Look at both mother and child. Is he sick or well? Is he normal or abnormal? Does he resemble his parents? Always look at children without staring or looking too closely at them. Some toddlers share attributes with certain animals who do not like being stared at. Any instinc-

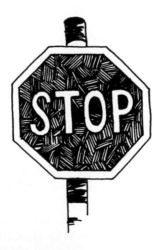

Fig. 3.1 Stop!

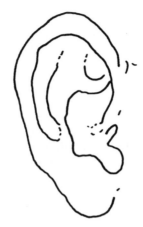

Fig. 3.2 Listen!

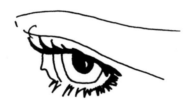

Fig. 3.3 Look!

tual clues? One must teach students to observe. Any observational cues?

Learn to see things.

Leonardo da Vinci

The approach code
Stop
Listen
Look
Use your other senses

Children are best approached in *their* position of comfort – lying flat in infancy, sitting on their mother's knee in toddler-hood, on their own two feet when of school age. Leave undressing to later – removal of clothes can be a threatening manoeuvre. Explain what you are about to do and be reassuring repeatedly. Don't lie the child down until you have to – he's very vulnerable in this position. Keep his mother close at hand. Always leave unpleasant procedures – throat examination, rectal examination – until the very last and don't do unless you feel they will be contributory.

Learn by listening to mothers, examining their children and then reading the chart. Too often students first read the notes and then go in search of what they are supposed to find. Students should at times take the opportunity of divesting their white coats – white coats bring needles and tests.

Never examine the presenting part only. From your earliest days train yourself to be thorough, and to be a generalist as opposed to a systems specialist. Remember one of the basic axioms – the good doctor treats the whole person, not just the sore belly or foot.

In summary, the best approach to infants and toddlers is to begin examination with a *strict no touch technique*. Be a good looker.

Look with all your eyes, look!

Jules Verne

In small infants *inspection* (of colour, breathing, activity, etc.) can be the key to diagnosis. Physical signs are frequently less florid in sick infants than they are in sick adults; students tend to be well trained in the arts of palpation and percussion, at the expense of inspection. We would agree with the words of Sir Dominic Corrigan (1853): 'The trouble with many doctors is not that they do not know enough but that they do not see enough.' Remember the importance of non-verbal communication. When you have looked, describe what you see. It is strange how difficult it can be to translate the observations into words. To say for example 'funny looking kid' (a pejorative term, objectionable to some) without being able to describe what is 'funny' is ludicrous. The road to diagnosis in many dermatological problems is to set down in words (of English or literate Latin) what one sees. All too often the descriptive terms elude the student and he jumps at diagnoses like a salmon at flies.

Syndrome spotting is in the eye and mental computer of the beholder. Students need not be syndrome spotters. However, they should be able to recognize Down's syndrome, obvious congenital abnormalities, or significant dysmorphism.

First know the normal. Then the abnormal or different may become apparent. Ask yourself, 'What's odd about this face?' Then describe in simple terms those relevant features – wide eyes, low-set ears, upturned nose, arched palate – which contribute to your suspicions.

You should try to examine as much with your eyes as with your hands. You should also try to listen to the child 'speaking with his body' – noting that many childhood physical complaints have a background behavioural basis.

Use your other senses – touch, smell, taste (occasionally) – to aid in diagnosis. These we will expand upon later. The child's doctor needs to be gentle of touch (cold hands-warm heart theorizing just will not do), to be able to extemporize (in other words to do what you can when you can and not to adhere to a rigid, regimented approach to examination), but to be thoroughly sensitive and sensible.

It will be frequently necessary to humour the baby or to distract an infant's attention when attempting examination. The **distraction tricks** (common sense really!) described below may help:

- play with babies, infants and children
- tickle babies (tickles appear at 3 months)
- play 'peek-a-boo'
- blow 'raspberries' at babies
- blow on their faces (they quite like this)
- allow toddlers to play with the examining instruments
- give infants something to hold
- get mother to dangle an attractive toy or bright light
- talk nonsense/rubbish to young children – they've quite a good sense of humour and may think you're a likeable idiot.

You can do anything with children if you only play with them.

Otto von Bismarck (19th century)

Shake hands with children: curiously, even toddlers may appreciate this formality. Hopefully you have allowed him

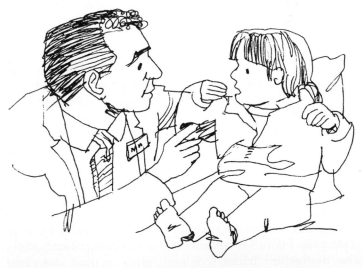

Fig. 3.4 Establish good eye contact and rapport with the child.

to establish eye contact with you; social sensory contact may facilitate you in applying your examining hands. In other words, before you start, try to strike a rapport.

Before proceeding to discuss detailed physical examination of different ages and various parts of children, we would remind you of the four Cs of clinical examination which you should aim to achieve:

- confidence   – of child in you (and you in yourself)
- competence   – in handling children
- completeness – of examination
- collation   – can you sum up and draw conclusions from what you've found?

THINGS NOT TO DO

Do not get the *gender* of the child wrong. This is understandably upsetting to parents. They begin to wonder if it is their child you are talking about. Never refer to a child as 'it'. This is a frequent failing, sure to raise the ire of certain colleagues and examiners.

Never handle a child *roughly*. Gentleness must be the hallmark of a good child's doctor. Apley used to preach: 'It's my fault if the child cries.' One need not go as far as this, but must attempt not to cause distress during physical examination.

Do not speak derogatively in front of children. Even little ears are more attuned to doctors' talk than you may think. Never refer to a child as an 'FLK' (funny looking kid) in front of the parents or without first seeing the parents. The term 'dysmorphic' might be more appropriate.

Do not drop the baby; they can be slippery, wriggly creatures especially if covered in vernix caseosa. Our experience of a student dropping a baby (fortunately without

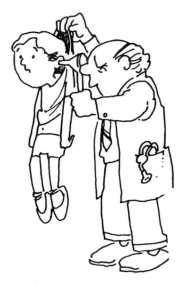

Fig. 3.5 Don't handle children roughly.

harm) when demonstrating the Moro reflex to examiners was salutary.

Do not use *potentially worrying terms* in front of parents without explaining them. The term 'pyloric tumour' may seem innocuous to you. However, to the layman, tumour implies cancer. Similarly, we have given the diagnosis 'benign recurrent haematuria' to parents with explanation and reassurance, without realizing that some of them had interpreted the word 'benign' to imply that the urinary blood was coming from a benign cancer of the kidney. It is often prudent to tell parents of children who are anaemic, 'Of course, it's not leukaemia'. Fear of cancer lurks in many a parental mind, at times and on occasions when it never occurs to their attending doctors.

Do not misjudge the child's *age* – children are remarkably sensitive on this score. Better to overestimate than to underestimate age.

Do not disrespect the child's intrinsic *modesty* – which will vary between and within societies. Some children will not mind being fully undressed; others may need explanation or a compromise.

POINT TO THE PART WHICH HURTS

Pain is a common reason for paediatric consultation. Clearly the bulk of the history concerning pain will be sought from the parents. However, you must always ask the child to try to describe *his* pain.

The preschool child will certainly lack the vocabulary and communication skills to describe his pains, but can surely point them out. So ask him to show you the spot which hurts. He can often pinpoint the appropriate place.

The older child should be asked to describe his pain, always checking with the parent his accuracy and veracity. A good mother will frequently coax the child without being asked: 'It's your pain, try to tell the doctor about it'.

Where is the pain?
Show me where it is?
What is it like?
What do you do when you get it?
Does it make you cry?

If the child can point to the spot, this should be reflected in your notes – 'left temporal headache' rather than just 'headache', or 'pain both upper thighs at night' rather than merely 'limb pains'.

A toddler or preschool child may resist abdominal examination. In the first instance distraction techniques

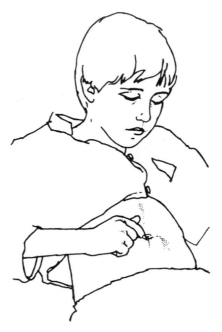

Fig. 3.6 Ask the child to point to the part which hurts.

may be tried. If these fail, use the child's hand to guide yours around the abdomen. A fretful child may allow you to assess abdominal pain or tenderness in this fashion.

One not infrequently meets the child with recurrent abdominal pain who is 'jumpy' and who seems to demonstrate tenderness on palpation, especially in the right iliac fossa. If in doubt as to the significance of this 'tenderness' a useful ploy is to say, 'I'm just going to listen with my stethoscope'. Lay it gently on the abdomen and do indeed listen but gradually increase the pressure. Often, quite firm pressure can be tolerated where previously there was 'tenderness'.

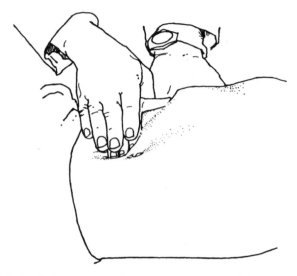

Fig. 3.7 Small children may allow you to palpate the abdomen over their own hand.

The child whose pain moves about in erratic fashion, crossing anatomical boundaries and disobeying dermatomes, needs to be taken with a grain of salt. Conversely, the child whose pain wakes him from his sleep, disturbs pleasurable activities or causes him to cry needs to be heeded.

Unwillingness to move or use a limb may suggest pain therein. Dislike of being handled is typical of meningism. Pleuritic pain may be evident by splinting of only one side of the chest – which is an infrequent, subtle sign missed even by experienced paediatricians. Small children have similarities with pets – when sick or sore they lie down without having to be told to do so.

The only time children tell the truth is when they are in pain.
Bill Cosby

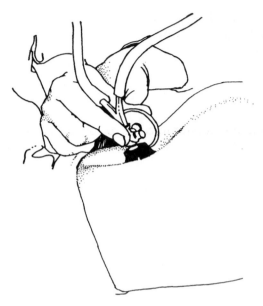

Fig. 3.8 Using the stethoscope to assess abdominal tenderness.

We don't agree entirely with the above statement, but do accept the sentiment that childhood pain is not figmentary.

PUTTING IT TOGETHER

Insofar as undergraduate students are concerned, diagnosis per se is not important. What is important is the ability to take a thorough history, elicit the relevant physical signs following examination, and attempt to interpret them. On the basis of the history and physical findings, the student may be able to construct a diagnosis, or a series of possible diagnoses.

Students must be prepared to write down their findings for public scrutiny. One can afford to be wrong as a student and learn from these mistakes. Being wrong may be a dent to one's doctoring dignity once qualified – in our opinion we should be more often prepared to say, 'I don't know, but I'll look it up'. Students could usefully cultivate the practice of writing down things they don't understand, or findings whose explanation is unclear (for example: What is the physiology of yawning?), and of seeking the answers.

One should attempt to come to conclusions on the completion of history and physical examination. For example:

Problems

1. Febrile convulsion
2. Follicular tonsillitis
3. Innocent murmur.

It may be useful to add a postscript:

Mother's worries

1. Brain damage
2. Nephew died of meningitis

and to deal with these prior to discharge.

If less sure of one's conclusions the 'bottom line' may read:

Impression

1. Failure to thrive
2. Possible anaemia
3. Consider malabsorption.

Note: Small, poor parents, no previous measurements.

It should be stated that differential diagnosis tends to play a less important part in paediatrics than in adult medicine, in that many childhood illnesses are straightforward uncomplicated entities compared with the complicated, cumulative, degenerative conditions of adulthood. Nonetheless one may have to consider and construct a differential diagnosis for diffuse lymphadenopathy, polyarthritis, acute encephalopathy, ataxia, haematuria, and many other clinical conditions.

Today's computer-literate students may like the key word approach: writing down the important positive findings plus relevant negative findings and attempting to compute an answer:

erythematous rash
Raynaud's phenomenon
pauciarticular arthritis
alopecia
weight loss
swollen parotid gland.

The above example suggests a connective tissue disorder.

In recording the physical findings of children with multiple or chronic disorders, the problem-based approach has much to recommend it. Table 3.1 shows an example from the notes of a child with spina bifida.

The list could be extended further, but we hope you have got the message. Detection and diagnosis of problems

Table 3.1 Example of a problem-based approach	
Problem	Plan
Myelomeningocele	Repaired after birth
Hydrocephalus, ventriculoperitoneal shunt	Check function
Moderate scoliosis	Physiotherapy, posture
Constipation	Discuss diet, nursing
Urinary incontinence	Self-catheterization?
Short stature	No action
Lower limb paralysis	Physiotherapy, walking devices

is only useful if it can lead to a plan of action for their improvement.

I DON'T KNOW

Teach thy tongue to say:

> I do not know.

Maimonides (1135–1204)

Doctors like to surround themselves with an aura of omniscience (how many doctors will consult a text in front of patients?). Students are not expected to know everything. If asked a question of which you don't know the answer, be prepared to say so rather than hazarding guesses. But you must later be prepared to look for the answer, solution or information or to ask the appropriate people to help you in finding out.

A constantly questioning mind will serve you well during your career. The back pages of this text could well be filled with questions seeking answers. Above all don't be shy in asking. Simple questions often provide fascinating answers.

DIAGNOSTIC LOGIC

The purpose of consultation between doctors and parents of sick children is to establish the cause of their concerns, to reach, if possible, a diagnosis and to formulate a plan of appropriate investigation and management. Diagnosis is essentially a process of deductive logic.

The history, properly taken, establishes facts. Productive histories will depend on attentive listening and knowing when and where to ask the salient questions.

The physical examination, properly conducted, should produce the findings. The facts and findings are collated and hopefully clinical reasoning will suggest a diagnosis or a differential diagnosis. This entails considering and weighing the relevant facts and findings, or producing a problem list. The good student excels by the ability to summarize and synthesize the critical information gleaned from clinical consultation.

We often, in our clinics, ask students:

- Have you formed an impression of the problem(s) presented?
- Can you summarize the key problem?
- Are you approaching a definite diagnosis?
- Can you hypothesize a differential diagnosis and weigh the evidence?

Think of the critical information you would need to collect to answer the following clinical scenarios:

- 7-year-old child still bed-wetting
- 8-year-old girl with early breast development
- toddler with multiple forehead bruises
- 2-year-old child with only monosyllables.

The good diagnostician picks up the alerting cues and clues, asks probing questions, and thinks logically: an amalgam of common sense, instinct, experience and observation.

> Observe, record, tabulate, communicate, use your five senses.
>
> William Osler

The well child is lively, a good colour, interactive, usually obliging and able to perform all of your clinical requests promptly and reliably. Well children will be seen for examination in general practitioner clinics, at child welfare clinics, and at school medicals. Do please practise examination of well children when permitted!

SYNDROME RECOGNITION

Undergraduate medical students do *not* need to be experts on recognizing syndromes and major congenital malformations, but they ought to initiate the fundamentals in rec-

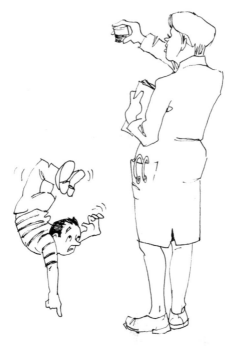

Fig. 3.9 An obviously well child.

ognizing and describing dysmorphic infants and children. Let's start with Down's syndrome, the most frequent chromosomal abnormality seen in paediatric practice. The secret is to describe what you see, pick up the cues, and assemble the key words:

- small head
- round face
- epicanthic folds
- protruding tongue
- short stature
- anteverted nose

- transverse palmar creases
- stubby fingers
- short fifth finger
- hypotonia
- delayed motor and cognitive development
- many associated medical problems.

The other trisomies, Edwards and Patau's syndromes, are rarely seen in children's wards since early demise is the norm.

Turner's syndrome, by contrast, is much more subtle. The classic textbook example of XO syndrome (neck webbing, wide nipples, lymphoedema of hands and feet, short stature) is not that commonly seen and many examples of Turner's syndrome may be XX/XO mosaics or other chromosomal variations.

Students spending some of their paediatric rotation in a tertiary centre may see children with mucopolysaccharidoses (Hurler's + variants), chromosome 22 deletion syndrome (cardiofacial syndrome), fetal alcohol syndrome and examples of achondroplasia. All that is expected of undergraduate students is an attempt to describe the dysmorphisms, an initial ability to assemble key words, and a basic idea of where next to consult. Computer-literate students may know of OMIM (Online Mendelian Inheritance in Man) or their library may possess the London Dysmorphology Database or Australian POSSUM programme. The best reference text is *Smith's Recognizable Patterns of Human Malformation*.

A deceased dysmorphology colleague used to ask students: 'How do you recognize your Aunt Molly?' *Answer*: 'Because you've seen her before'! A good look, a little knowledge and a programmed computer is all that undergraduate students require. Postgraduate students and paediatric trainees will be expected to develop their clinical skills, prime their senses, and progressively recognize paediatric syndromes with experience and maturation.

4 Examination at different ages

Paediatrics is a specialty bound by age and not by system.

Apley

NEWBORN

The great majority of newborn infants have had a normal intrauterine existence, a normal delivery, are in good condition at birth and are physically normal. However, there is a considerable variation in size and shape and appearance within the normal, which depends on parental, familial, genetic and ethnic factors. The foundation stone of paediatric medicine is only laid when the student has personally examined a large number of normal neonates, infants, toddlers, preschool and older children. The message, therefore, is: know the normal spectrum.

Delivery room

All newborns should be examined at birth to observe the general condition and to rule out major anomalies. The Apgar score (Table 4.1) is valuable because it determines whether resuscitation is necessary or not, and it is internationally accepted. A poor score (<5) at 5 minutes appears to relate to long-term development. Examination of the cord for a single artery may be of some value as to the possibility of as yet hidden abnormalities. Having established that the baby does not require special or intensive care, and is overtly normal, the parents are accordingly informed.

Postnatal ward

A further examination is usually carried out on the third day, at which time the baby is almost unrecognizable from the one examined at delivery – skin nice and pink, head assuming normal shape, hair combed and feeding well. The examination at this stage is much more detailed. The mother,

Table 4.1 Apgar score			
Sign	Score		
	0	1	2
Colour	Blue, pale	Pink trunk Blue extremities	Pink all over
Heart rate	Absent	<100	> 100
Reflex irritability	None	Grimace	Cry
Tone, activity	Limp	Some limb flexion	Active movement
Respiratory effort	Absent	Slow, irregular	Good strong cry

and, if possible, the father should be present. Explanation should be offered as the examination proceeds and each test described as it is being performed. The mother is particularly influenced by the appearance of her baby: include size (is he in normal centiles?), facial appearance, colour and texture of skin, bruising, abrasions, scratch marks, rashes and subconjunctival haemorrhage. The latter condition is easily understood if the mother has suffered the same as a result of labour.

Blotchy erythematous rash is common; this is almost certainly erythema toxicum. Peeling of the skin that has been exposed to meconium is normal. This can be confirmed by discolouration of the cord stump and the presence of stained fingernails. Fingernails are often long and although soft can cause scratch marks. The toenails often appear to be ingrowing and this is of no consequence.

Jaundice is best observed in the sclera, skin and mucous membranes, preferably in good daylight. Always switch off phototherapy unit lights when attempting to determine jaundice. We believe that it remains good practice (although fallible) to attempt to determine the degree of jaundice clinically but always measure serum bilirubin of jaundiced babies. Phototherapy can induce the 'bronzed baby' syndrome.

Head and face

As the appearance of the baby is of concern to the mother, inspection and examination of the head and face should be carried out first. Local trauma is common and includes caput succedaneum and moulding, minor abrasions of the scalp, forceps marks, non-specific facial bruises, subconjunctival haemorrhage and occasionally cephalhaematoma. In general, these conditions resolve spontaneously within the first week with the notable exception of

53

cephalhaematoma, which will calcify and resolve within 2–3 months. Cephalhaematoma is most commonly found over the parietal bone and confined to the edges. Occasionally both parietal bones are involved. Rarely the condition can involve the occipital bone when the possibility of an encephalocele should be considered.

Asymmetry of the face may occasionally be due to a transient 7th cranial nerve paresis, which nearly always results from a forceps delivery. Head shape varies considerably during the first week. Marked moulding with caput occurs in some. Intrauterine pressure (when the fetus is in breech position) may produce an elongated head with protuberance of the occiput. Deflection, giving rise to face presentation, may be associated with severe bruising and oedema of the face, eyelids and lips. Chvostek's sign (tapping the facial nerve → twitching of the perioral muscles) is a normal finding in the newborn.

Plagiocephaly is not an uncommon finding related to intrauterine position. The head is skewed slightly or noticeably. The simple trick of placing one finger in each ear of the forward-looking head will demonstrate plagiocephaly readily.

The anterior fontanelle is normally open and can vary from 1 cm to 4 or 5 cm in diameter. Cranial sutures are usually mobile and the posterior fontanelle may accept a fingertip.

Ears

Ears can be of different shape and size and the amount of cartilage can vary. A low-set ear where the top of the pinna is below a horizontal line from the outer canthus does not make a syndrome. Nor does the presence of preauricular ear tags.

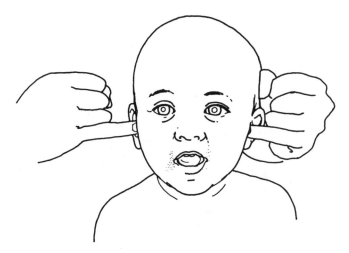

Fig. 4.1 Demonstrating plagiocephaly in the older infant.

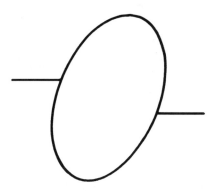

Fig. 4.2 Plagiocephaly.

Mouth

The shape of the mouth varies and a slanting lower jaw only reflects intrauterine head posture. Look for presence of a tooth, examine gums anteriorly and posteriorly to exclude ranula or cyst, check the size and shape of tongue.

The lingual frenum extends from the undersurface of the tongue to the floor of the mouth and is present in all children. Surgery on the frenum may rarely be required if there is interference with tongue protrusion or with growth of tongue tip. The soft palate and uvula should be observed.

Come to terms: head

frontal bossing = prominence of forehead, i.e. part of frontal bone
craniotabes   = soft compressible skull bones

Come to terms: skull shapes

scaphocephaly = boat-shaped head (long, narrow)
macrocephaly = large head (synonym = megalencephaly)
microcephaly = very small head
plagiocephaly = parallelogram (skew) head
turricephaly   = tall head (synonym = acrocephaly)
brachycephaly = flat head (short head)
synostosis   = premature fusion of adjacent bones
trigonocephaly = triangular-shaped head

Eyes

Oedema of the eyelids is common, more particularly in the preterm baby. Bruising may also be present. Because of the oedema, opening the eyes may be difficult; if the examiner holds the baby in the upright or prone position, in most cases the eyes open. Look for conjunctival haemorrhage, clear cornea, evidence of cataract. Compare eye size and if in doubt palpate the eyes for size and eyeball pressure.

Squint is common, although rarely paralytic, in which case the 6th cranial nerve is usually involved. Accumulation of lacrimal fluid with secondary infection is extremely common and results usually from incomplete drainage of the nasolacrimal duct. If there is a lot of pus present, a specific infection such as gonococcal ophthalmia should be considered.

Respiratory system

The respiratory system is best examined by observation. Observation of the colour of the baby's lips, mucosa and skin, and observation of respiratory rate and effort is infinitely more important than percussion or auscultation. Observation should include the rate of respiration (normally 30–50 per minute at rest), the rhythm of respiration and the work of respiration. Normal newborn respiration is quiet, effortless and predominantly diaphragmatic. There is more abdominal than chest movement.

Respiratory problems are common in the newborn and will be manifest by tachypnoea, increased respiratory effort and cyanosis. The baby may develop retraction, recession and variable respiratory rhythm. The student should comment on chest shape and outline and use of accessory muscles of respiration.

Come to terms: respiration

tachypnoea	= respiratory rate > 60 per minute
sternal retraction	= insuction of sternum in inspiration
intercostal recession	= excessive indrawing of intercostal muscles during respiration
periodic breathing	= alternating rhythm of respiration with periods of apnoea (common in preterms)

Cardiovascular system

At the outset observe colour, respiratory effort, shape of chest, precordial bulge and/or heave. Localization of the trachea and the apex beat is important. The position of the apex beat may be difficult to localize but usually is between the 4th and 5th space in the midclavicular line. Precordial thrills are not uncommon in the newborn and should always be sought. Palpation of the brachial and femoral pulse may require total concentration, bearing in mind that too much pressure may obliterate it. The best advice is repetitive practice.

The heart sounds should be listened to at both the apex and base, commenting on the first sound at the apex and the second sound at the base. Not uncommonly a physiological third heart sound may be heard. The heart rate varies from 100 to 140 per minute. Occasionally extrasystoles may be noted and usually are of no significance. Heart block without a structural anomaly of the heart is extremely rare and can be diagnosed antenatally.

Systolic murmurs are common and usually best heard along the left sternal border. A short high-pitched localized murmur which is not transmitted is generally benign and in the absence of any other positive finding a diagnosis of innocent murmur is made. As a precaution this should be rechecked before discharge and again at 3 and 6 weeks. The student should only be concerned with systolic murmurs in this age group. Listen to as many as possible – examine, examine, examine! With practice and in older babies you may pick up diastolic murmurs as the heart rate is slower.

Abdomen

Again, first observe. The abdomen is often generally somewhat distended – more so after a feed (so enquire!).

Respiration is reflected in abdominal movement via the diaphragm and this is normal. If in doubt about distension measure at a marked point above or below the umbilicus. Observe the umbilicus. Is it ageing normally – any blood or discharges? Is there a smell? Is there periumbilical inflammation? Is the umbilical vein visible? Is it inflamed? Reassure mother that the cord will part spontaneously around the fourth or fifth day. Is there any evidence of an early umbilical hernia? Occasionally palpation of the abdomen may cause the baby to regurgitate mucus or feed. So be very careful.

Palpate the abdomen gently (with the aid of a soother if necessary). Use your right hand to examine for the spleen, whose tip is often readily palpable. It does not matter from which side you approach the examination of a newborn abdomen – just be comfortable. Check the liver edge by placing your palm between the umbilicus and right iliac crest. Get the feel of the abdomen and then slowly proceed towards the rib cage. Remember that the right lobe of the liver is what you are going to meet first. The liver edge is usually soft and easily missed. It is nearly always palpable up to 2–3 cm below the costal margin. There is little doubt that the kidneys in the average newborn can be palpated, particularly the lower poles. However, this is not easy and requires considerable practice. The most suitable method is to place one hand under the upper lumbar region, exerting gentle pressure upwards while doing the actual palpation with the other hand. The examiner is trying to establish the presence of both kidneys and whether or not they are enlarged.

The bladder (when full) is an abdominal organ in the newborn and is best felt approximately 15 minutes after a feed. Starting just below the umbilicus using the index and second finger and thumb, gently feel for the bladder, gradually moving pincer grasp downwards until felt. When a bladder is palpable, gentle massage will produce a contraction, following which a midstream specimen can be obtained without contamination. A large bladder is frequently noted where the infant has asphyxial encephalopathy or a severe neural tube defect.

Note that inguinal lymph nodes are often palpable in the newborn and are a normal finding.

Genitalia

Female. Labia may be quite red and minora not covered, particularly in the preterm. Labial fusion is sometimes present and is easily dealt with if required. Vaginal tags are common and should be ignored. They will resolve spontaneously during the first week. Vaginal haemorrhage ('newborn period') occasionally occurs. Bruising may be present, particularly if the baby had a breech delivery. Increased pigmentation and enlargement of the clitoris should be noted. *Male.* Is the penis of normal size and shape? Is there any evidence of hypospadias? (Epispadias is exceedingly rare.) Hypospadias is commonly glandular (or coronal), infrequently in the shaft (penile), and rarely at the base (perineal). Are the testes palpable and of normal size? If testes are not in the scrotum, commence in the inguinal area and palpate downwards. If a testis appears bigger than average, consider hydrocele (common) and confirm by transillumination. There may be an associated inguinal hernia, which is more common in males, particularly in the preterm. Very rarely an enlarged testis may be due to torsion; the testis then feels hard and is discoloured.

Musculo-skeletal system

The examination of bones, joints, ligaments and the attached muscles is of fundamental importance in the newborn.

Dislocatable (loose) hips

The term developmental dysplasia of the hips (DDH) has replaced the term congenital dislocation of the hips. Clinical examination for dislocated or dislocatable hips is not entirely reliable. Ultrasonic screening is used to augment clinical examination.

True dislocation is rare at birth, with the notable exception of the baby with severe neural tube defect (meningomyelocele). Unstable hip, however, is common and occurs in approximately 15–20 per 1000 live births. This condition is extremely uncommon in the preterm. Overall, unstable hip is more common in the female except following breech presentation where the risk is equal in both sexes. Talipes calcaneo valgus may also be associated with it. The left hip is twice as likely to be involved as the right hip.

The earlier the hip examination is carried out the better. Day 1 is now the day of choice with the best chance of positive diagnosis. In general, Barlow's method of examination

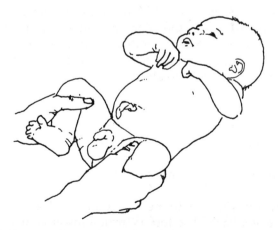

Fig. 4.3 Examining hips in the newborn baby.

is preferred. It is important that the baby is placed on a flat table (approximately waist high from the examiner), in the supine position and if possible relaxed. Position the hips and knees at 90° and grasp both knees between thumb and index and second fingers, the tips of which are over the outer trochanter of each femur. Press the hips gently backwards and then abduct and lift with the outside fingers – if the hip is loose a clunking feeling is noted when lifting the head of the femur back into the socket. The gentler this test is performed the better the response. It is important to be gentle when carrying out this test and it certainly should not be done repetitively. It is very easy to damage the hip joint. Total abduction of the hip joint should never be carried out during physical examination.

Ortolani's (relocation) test. Ortolani's test relocates a dislocated hip into the joint. The click/clunk is caused by the head crossing the acetabulum. One way to remember it is:

$$\underline{O}RTOLAN\underline{I} = O, I \ (out \rightarrow in)$$

Please remember that Barlow's and Ortolani's tests can only be performed in the neonatal period. By age 6 weeks these manoeuvres are unproductive because of increased muscle tone. After 6 weeks the only reliable clinical test for dislocation is limited hip abduction.

Feet

Mobility of the foot joints is the major factor determining the need for treatment or non-treatment. Deformities of the foot are common and vary in type.

Tarsus varus. This is extremely common – a degree occurs in nearly every baby. The foot is turned inwards to a varying degree at the tarsal joints. Spontaneous recovery is the rule, although occasionally transient manipulation and massage may be necessary.

Calcaneo valgus. This condition is also common and appears to occur more often in the post term and may occasionally be associated with a loose hip. The dorsum of the foot is in a position close to the shin. As calf muscle tone improves, the foot is pulled into the normal position; this usually occurs within 6–8 weeks.

Talipes equino varus (primary club foot). This condition occurs in 1 per 1000 births and is twice as common in the male baby. In 50% of cases it is bilateral. Usually there is a fixed structural deformity with involvement of both the fore- and hindfoot and associated wasting of the calf muscles. Early manipulation and fixation is advisable.

Other minor anomalies of the toes occur, including over-riding (usually 3rd or 4th) and overlapping of the 5th toe. Toenails always appear ingrowing in the newborn – this is a normal phenomenon. Treatment is usually not required for any of these conditions.

Minor variants not minor anomalies:

- mild to moderate bowing of lower leg
- mild syndactyly of 2nd and 3rd toes
- shallow sacral dimple
- hydrocele of testes
- single upper palmar crease.

Spine

Examination of the spinal processes should be carried out with the baby lying in the prone position and palpating each spinal process. Occasionally a spina bifida occulta or dermal sinus may be noted. More often a postanal dimple is present; this is of no consequence (Table 4.2), and the parents should be reassured.

Table 4.2 Types of congenital malformation

System	Major	Minor
Craniofacial	Cleft lip/palate Sutural synostosis	Plagiocephaly
Abdominal	Exomphalos/ Gastroschisis	Umbilical hernia
Spinal	Neural tube defect	Sacral dimple
Foot	Talipes equino varus	2–3 toe syndactyly

Central nervous system

Examination of this system in the newborn is entirely different from that of the older child. It is the assessment of posture and tone, movement and primitive reflexes. Therefore, much information may be obtained (once again) by spending a few minutes observing the infant. In general, the posture is entirely flexor although abnormal intrauterine posture can distort this: for example, extended breech or deflexed head. The complete flexor posture is not fully adopted until 37 completed weeks. Observe limb movements – are they normal? There is a great variation ranging from tremulous movements of one or all limbs to jittery movements, both of which may be normal. Feel the upper and lower limbs, establish flexor recoil and compare. If doubt exists then the examination should be repeated with the head held in the midline. Having the 'posture-picture', proceed to assess tone by doing the *neck traction test*. Here hands are firmly grasped and the infant is pulled to the sitting position. The head should flex and follow the traction to upright position and hold momentarily. This is an important test (see Fig. 4.4).

Vertical suspension is assessed by grasping the infant under each axilla. The normal baby supports himself in this position. The term baby who slips through suggests hypotonia.

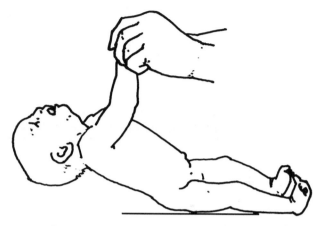

Fig. 4.4 Neck traction.

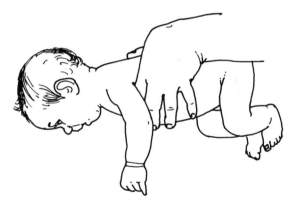

Fig. 4.5 Ventral suspension.

Ventral suspension is assessed by placing the baby prone on the palm of the hand. In the normal response the back extends, arms and knees flex, hips extend and head lifts and rotates.

Lower limb posture in the supine position is usually flexor with the hips slightly abducted. Full abduction of the hips in a supine term baby indicates hypotonia and is abnormal.

It must be stressed that when one or more of these tests suggest hypotonia a repeat examination in 24 hours may confirm or otherwise the significance of the previous examination. Remarkable changes in tone and posture can occur in a matter of hours during the first week of life.

Deep tendon reflexes can be readily elicited – particularly the knee tendon reflex. Flex the particular joint and hold the limb with the same hand and tap tendon with fingertip. Intermittent ankle clonus may also be present in the normal baby and is detected by gentle but sudden dorsiflexion of the foot.

Pointers to hypotonia

- Head lag
- Slips through on upright suspension
- Like 'rag doll' in ventral suspension
- Total hip abduction.

Primitive reflexes

A number of primitive reflexes are present and easily elicited in the normal term baby. These gradually disappear and are not present at the end of the sixth month with the notable exception of the blink response, which remains. Do these tests properly since the best response is usually obtained on the first test. The response tends to wane on repeated testing.

Blink response. A gentle tap above the nasal bridge usually evokes the blink response. This test is nearly always normal except in the very ill baby.

Cardinal signs. These collectively refer to sensory stimulation of the cheek and skin around the mouth and lips. Pressing a finger on the cheek near the mouth and moving it laterally will cause the baby to open his mouth and turn the head to root for a nipple. When a soother or nipple is placed in the mouth, the normal baby will suck vigorously (depending somewhat on the timing of the previous feed) and swallow in unison.

Grasp and traction response. This has been referred to previously in relation to tone. This test, however, can be

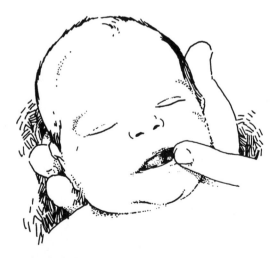

Fig. 4.6 Cardinal points.

provoked unilaterally by placing a finger or pencil in the baby's palm. This causes grasping and with gentle upward traction the forearm and shoulder muscles will contract. When carried out properly the infant may be lifted 2–3 cm from the surface of the cot. When the baby is lowered, gentle stroking of the ulnar surface of the palm will disengage the grasp.

To record an optimal response in the following tests it is preferable that the baby's head is in the midline.

Asymmetrical tonic neck reflex. This test may easily be elicited by leaving the infant lying in the supine position and slowly turning the head 90° to the right and left. The upper and lower limbs extend on the facial side and, similarly, there is flexion on the occipital side, producing the classic sword fighting or fencing posture.

Moro reflex. This is the most widely known and frequently elicited test. The baby is laid supine on the forearm and

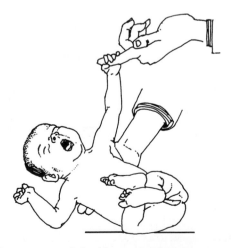

Fig. 4.7 Palmar grasp and shoulder traction response.

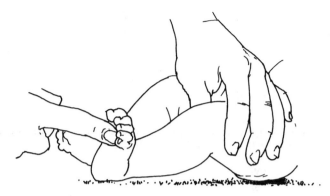

Fig. 4.8 Toe grasp.

hand and the head is held in the other hand. The response occurs when the head is 'dropped' a few centimetres. The upper limbs abduct, extend and flex in a flowing movement symmetrically; a poor or no response indicates a major problem. However, a unilateral response confirms the damage (usually transient) to the fifth and sixth cervical roots producing the classic Erb's paresis.

Spinal curve or Galant reflex. Hold the baby on one hand (similar to ventral suspension test) and stroke the lateral border of the spinal muscle from the mid-thoracic area downwards. This will cause the pelvis to curve to the same side. A similar response should be evoked on the opposite side.

Crossed extension reflex. While keeping the baby in the supine position, extend one knee and stroke the foot on the same side; this will cause the opposite leg to flex, abduct and extend 'to push away' the provoking hand.

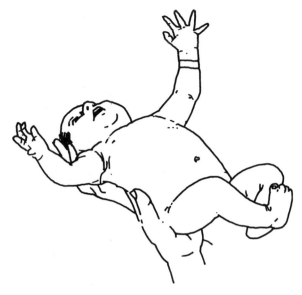

Fig. 4.9 Moro response.

Extensor thrust, placing and walking reflex. These movements relate and provide evidence of lower limb function. With the baby held between both hands, the legs lowered to the surface, pressure on the soles of the feet may cause the lower limbs to suddenly extend, producing an extensor thrust. If the lower limbs, with the baby still held in the same position, are pressed against the edge of the examining table one foot will flex to place. By bringing the baby's limbs further on to the table leaning forwards at an angle of 10–20° a walking movement may be produced.

Hearing. A crude hearing response can certainly be elicited in the newborn. The simplest test is to say 'aaah' into the crying baby's ear from a distance of 3–4 cm. Usually this

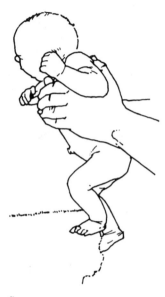

Fig. 4.10 Placing reflex.

produces a cessation of crying. A startle response to a loud noise may be a crude indicator of hearing. Specific screening tests are now available.

Vision. The newborn can see and will readily turn to a light source. The infant may, for example, turn his head to the room or cubicle window. Also, when seated comfortably and with the baby held in the supine facing the examiner at an angle of about 30°, eye fixation can be established at a distance of about 20 cm. A red ball of 5–6 cm in diameter can be brought slowly across the baby's visual field, at which time following may occur. These latter tests require time, a cooperative baby and a certain expertise. Positive responses to vision and hearing tests are very reassuring to the mother.

Conclusion

Examination of the central nervous system in the newborn requires attention to detail, a deal of patience and a baby in the right mood. The value of transient alteration of one, two or even three tests is as yet not precisely clear. However, much research has and is being carried out in this area and there is little doubt that diligent and repetitive examination can be both rewarding and educational. The record of such a detailed examination may be of vital importance to the developmental paediatrician in later years.

Newborn examination: purposes	
Day 1	1. to assess general condition
	2. to establish normality
	3. to detect major abnormalities
Days 3–5 (discharge)	1. to confirm normality
	2. to detect minor abnormalities
	3. to assess neurological status

The preterm baby following discharge

As more very low birth weight and immature babies survive, they unfortunately can bring many clinical problems through to general paediatric medicine. Therefore, clinical and developmental assessment should target suspect areas specific to such children. In assessing development, allowance should be made for the duration of immaturity in weeks and also the extent and duration of serious illness during the postnatal period. As the child reaches 3–4 years this time factor becomes of little consequence.

In general, most babies of less than 30 weeks' gestation will have a long narrow-shaped head due to an initial inability to turn the head from side to side. This shape of head does not relate to developmental status. Emphasis in examination should be placed on head size (periventricular haemorrhage is common in infants less than 30 weeks) and the presence of a ventriculo-peritoneal shunt. Muscle tone and gross motor status may be less than optimum – mainly because of perinatal morbidity. Vision and fine movement and social behavioural assessment can give useful guidance to developmental quotient. Hearing impairment is not uncommon in the preterm infant. However, early more precise hearing tests are now available.

Retinopathy of some degree is common in the very immature but most infants will have had a thorough eye examination and treatment (laser) where required, prior to discharge. Overall, however, visual problems are common and assessment for strabismus should be detailed.

Bronchopulmonary dysplasia (BPD) commonly extends through the first and sometimes second year. Such infants are more prone to episodes of respiratory infections such as bronchiolitis. However, there is a gradual return to normal respiratory function. During clinical examination of such babies, tachypnoea at rest may be noted. Respiratory rate may also be influenced by the use of respiratory stimulant (theophylline) which some receive, particularly during the first year.

Umbilical hernias are commonly found but rarely require treatment. Inguinal hernias occur in approximately 25% of male preterm babies. Recognition of inguinal hernias is urgent as strangulation and obstruction may occur.

In general, gastrointestinal problems are uncommon. However, if the baby had necrotizing enterocolitis in the postnatal period then secondary disaccharide intolerance may result and in some cases strictures may cause problems.

Scarring of skin may be present due to drip sites, chest drains and particularly trauma from heel blood sampling.

Occasionally with prolonged tracheal intubation there may be alteration in the shape of the soft palate – this is referred to as a palatal groove. Capillary haemangiomas occur more commonly in the preterm baby. After an initial growth period, spontaneous regression can be expected in the first 2–5 years.

Although talipes equino varus (TEV) can occur in the preterm, developmental dysplasia of the hip is very uncommon. However, if there is a strong positive family history of hip dysplasia then further evaluation should be carried out during the first year, possibly including ultrasound examination.

SIX-WEEK EXAMINATION

The 6-week examination is an important postnatal event and all babies should be seen at this time.

The 6-week examination: purposes
1. to evaluate feeding pattern
2. to measure growth and weight gain
3. to detect abnormalities not noted in neonatal period
4. to assess early development
5. to ensure infant–maternal bonding

It is important at the 6-week assessment to have all the relevant perinatal details, including birth weight, head circumference and crown–heel length.

Measurement (centiles)

- Head circumference
- Length
- Weight.

Adverse perinatal history to note

- Asphyxia
- Low birth weight
- Preterm
- Infection
- Hypoglycaemia
- Trauma.

The process of examination should be careful and gentle. Take the fully dressed infant from his mother and lay him on a covered table. You should not allow the mother or nurse or anyone else to undress the infant. Do it yourself as the examination proceeds; get the feel of the baby yourself. Observe, without disturbing if possible. Look at the way the infant is dressed and the general picture of care. Look at the face – good colour, clean, no rash, scalp clear, normal quiet respiration or otherwise, any evidence of snuffles or noisy breathing? Is there any evidence of anaemia? Are the lips a good colour? Gently check the conjunctiva.

Feel the head and fontanelle, look for seborrhoea. If the infant is awake, try to get eye fixation from about 20 cm. Having achieved eye fixation often the baby will smile in return. Smiling with meaning is an important milestone. If, however, the infant is crying, say 'aaah' into his ear in low tone and crying may cease. If it does not, hold the infant upright and tip him forwards. Crying may cease and the eyes open. Then start again.

Now check head growth, feel the anterior fontanelle and sutures. Look for early head control. When holding the infant in the sitting position the head may fall forward but there should be reasonable, if wobbly, head control. Look at limb movements and check limb tone. Observe the hands – look for thumb abduction and finger flexion. If fisting is present, open the palm and observe for accumulation of dirt in the palmar creases. The skin of the palm may be moist and pale. This suggests the hands have been tightly clenched since birth. Look for persistent ankle clonus.

Check primitive reflexes, looking for accentuation of particularly the Moro, asymmetrical tonic neck and walking reflexes. Look at the state of nutrition, respiratory rate and general well-being. Is there any evidence of dehydration, loss of subcutaneous fat or wasting? Gently examine the mouth, particularly observing for evidence of monilial infection. Look for evidence of conjunctival infection. Roll tip of finger over inner canthus to clear lacrimal duct.

Transient blockage of nasolacrimal duct is very common. Check nose for snuffles – again an extremely common finding and usually of no serious consequence. Swelling of the infant's breasts may be present, and occasionally there is evidence of inflammation and abscess formation. Inflammation and infection of the corners of the fingernails and toenails (paronychia) are fairly common.

Developmental indicators	
frowning	3–6 weeks
smiling with meaning	5–8 weeks
early head control (5–10 s)	5–8 weeks
eye fixation on examination of face	6 weeks (20–30 cm)
vocalization (coo) may be present	6-week-old
(usually in a infant with siblings)	

Skin

Look for evidence of seborrhoea in the scalp and/or napkin dermatitis. Usually facial 'stork bite marks' are fading. Conversely, strawberry naevi become more defined and are growing. Port wine stain unfortunately becomes more defined as the skin becomes paler. Occasionally physiological jaundice may have persisted, particularly in association with breast feeding. However, the re-emergence of jaundice at 6 weeks is a sinister sign and must be thoroughly investigated.

Respiratory

Observe the infant's rate and type of breathing. Is it noisy? If so, what kind of noise – upper, lower, inspiratory or expiratory? Laryngomalacia is a common cause of inspiratory stridor in this age group. Coughing implies a lower respiratory infection – though specific abnormal sounds are rarely localized on auscultation.

Cardiovascular

Heart rate and pulses should be checked. The pulse will alter significantly if crying. Check the precordium and apex beat. Remember, a thrill is more easily felt in this age group. Listen to the heart sounds at the apex and also at the base, commenting on the first sound in the former and the second sound at the latter. Is there a murmur (which, with few notable exceptions, is nearly always systolic in nature)? Where is it best localized? Does it radiate? Is it loud? Is there a thrill? Most important of all, what is the duration and is it pansystolic? Try to decide if the murmur is significant or not.

Remember – a benign systolic murmur is short, high pitched, soft, not transmitted and there is no thrill. A venous hum (more common in toddlers) may be heard at the base. Pressure on the jugular vein should reduce this sound considerably.

Abdomen

Look at the shape. Is there any distension? Has the umbilicus healed completely? Is there any residual granulation tissue or is there any herniation? Palpate for the spleen, the tip of which may well be palpable. Feel the liver edge (2–3 cm) and percuss if necessary. Check for palpable bladder and perhaps lower poles of kidney. This latter examination becomes more difficult as the infants get older. Look at the genitalia. Are both testes palpable? Is there any evidence of hydrocele or inguinal hernia? Is there a reasonable preputial opening? In the female, check for labial fusion. Look at the anus, observe for blood staining and/or early fissure – a not uncommon problem.

Musculo-skeletal

In the majority the feet are normal, tarsus varus and calcaneo valgus having resolved spontaneously in the previous 4 weeks.

Examination of the hips is again important although much less rewarding than during the first week. Again use Barlow's test. One may find benign adductor spasm in some infants. Do not force the hips into full abduction as this manoeuvre can damage the hip joint. Subluxation at 6 weeks is rare.

The 6-week examination: 3 Hs and warning signals

3 Hs to highlight at 6 weeks

1. head: too big = ? hydrocephalus; too small = ? microcephaly
2. heart: murmurs may become apparent!
3. hips: test abduction

A thorough examination is from head to toe and is easy to do. Six-week-old babies and their mothers usually enjoy this examination.
Warning signals: 6 weeks

major maternal anxiety
unusually small or large head
hypotonia = poor ventral suspension, poor neck traction
persistent irritability
persistent thumb adduction

THE ACUTELY ILL INFANT

It is clear that further reductions in infant mortality will require doctors to sharpen their diagnostic wits and instincts. Infants have a very limited clinical vocabulary with which to express themselves and the identical symptoms (food refusal, vomiting, fever, lethargy) may reflect meningitis, pneumonia, or urinary tract infection.

Infants can become ill very rapidly – happily for the practising doctor they also recover promptly if appropriately treated. In infancy one must always heed the mother's judgement and opinion. We will now repeat the importance in approaching ill infants of:

• careful observation
• thorough examination
• instinctual suspicion.

Certain symptoms in infancy demand our immediate attention. Some of them are listed in the following box. Mothers will vary in their rapidity of response but most will recognize the seriousness of these complaints and seek help. Mothers in our country use the idiomatic expression 'he's not himself' to imply a significant change in their infant's well-being.

Always serious symptoms in infancy

High-pitched screaming or crying
Alternating drowsiness and irritability
Convulsion
Refusal to feed (two or more consecutive feeds)
Repeated vomiting
Rapid, laboured breathing, with or without grunting
Episodes of unusual blueness or paleness
Spreading purpuric spots >2 mm in diameter

Less serious symptoms, but ones not to be ignored, are detailed in the following box. Infants with these complaints will need to be kept under close observation. Croup is a source of great parental anxiety even though their infant may be apparently coping.

Usually serious symptoms in infancy
repeated diarrhoea prolonged crying croup (stridor, hoarseness, barking cough) high fever (40°C/104°F) persistent crankiness

One's first approach to the acutely and seriously ill infant is to observe the infant in his position of comfort. Note the heart rate, respiratory rate and effort, presence or absence of a rash, colour and temperature. Ill infants frequently have a mottled (or marbled) appearance to their skin. They lie still. Breathing is often rapid and grunting. The eyes have a glazed or distant look. They may be centrally warm and peripherally cold. They convulse easily with fever.

Note movement (or lack of it). Refusal to use a limb may suggest infection therein: for example, osteomyelitis. Splinting of the chest is occasionally seen in pneumonia. Arching of the neck occurs with meningitis. An immobile abdomen is very significant, appendicitis and peritonitis being notoriously difficult to detect in infancy.

One needs to make a statement about:

- degree of sickness
- hydration
- nutrition
- circulation.

Before proceeding to detailed examination, weight, temperature, pulse rate and respiratory rate will of course be recorded. Ill infants are usually fairly passive and can be examined in an organized fashion.

Degree of sickness

This can only be learned by experience and observation and not taught in texts or tutorials. So do spend time in the emergency room and admitting office. See and assess, regard and remember. Is he seriously ill? Is he moderately ill? Is he mildly ill?

Hydration

This can easily and rapidly be assessed (see p. 210). One wishes to determine if the infant is normally hydrated, dehydrated, or less commonly, overhydrated.

Nutrition

Nutrition can be quickly assessed by looking at and feeling subcutaneous fat, inspecting buttocks and muscle bulk, looking for lax skinfolds in the axilla and groin, and of course weighing the infant. Skinfold thickness and mid-arm circumference can be determined later if necessary. Is he plump, 'normal' or poorly nourished?

Circulation

What is his circulation like? Is the colour of tongue, lips, mucous membranes and nail beds normal? Is he mottled or cyanosed? Are the peripheries warm? Is capillary refill in the feet reasonably rapid? Warm toes (especially with palpable dorsalis pedis or posterior tibial pulse) are a reasonably good indicator of satisfactory circulatory state. One must not omit to measure blood pressure in acutely ill infants.

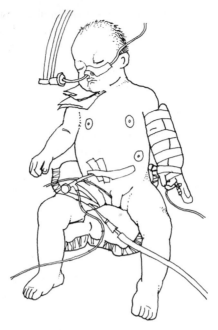

Fig. 4.11 The acutely ill infant.

Acute illness in infancy	
Medical sickness	**Surgical sickness**
meningitis	intussusception
pneumonia	appendicitis/peritonitis
osteomyelitis	intestinal obstruction
gastroenteritis	incarcerated hernia
septicaemia	
urinary tract infection	
croup syndromes	

Simple observations

Simply by looking at a baby or infant you can make some useful statements as for example:

normal infant
moderately ill
normally hydrated
well nourished
possibly anaemic
query respiratory tract infection.

Food refusal is a serious symptom in infancy. By contrast, the infant who feeds well may be ill, but not seriously so. We reassure mothers that their infants are reasonably well if they fulfil the 3 Fs:

good *form*
good *feeding*
no *fever*.

Think intussusception!

infant 6–12 months
acute episodes of pain with crying, drawing up of legs
extreme pallor
palpable abdominal mass
unexplained shock

THE TERRIFIED TODDLER

That enfant terrible of paediatrics, the toddler (1–3 years), warrants special mention. He can be clinging, resistive, screaming or downright impossible to examine. Approach him as you would any creature who feels he is cornered – slowly, carefully and with calculated caution. With experience and expertise you may be able to examine him surreptitiously and superficially. Do not remove him from his place of safety, his mother's knee, or embrace.

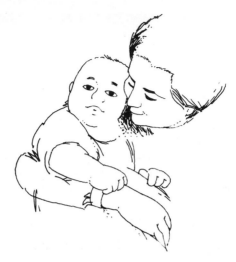

Fig. 4.12 Toddler in mother's arms – a safe examination position.

He does not like having his head circumference measured, his ear drums examined or his throat inspected; leave these until last. Give him toys (or even spatulae) to occupy both hands. Above all learn to be expedient and speedy in your examination. But don't rush him. The simple ploy of first placing your stethoscope on his knee may enable him to allow you to auscultate his heart.

One will always have to use one's wits and instincts in approaching the toddler. A lot can be achieved by examining him when asleep – you can observe colour, note rate and depth of respiration, palpate the pulse (e.g. preauricular), feel his skin temperature, see if he's coping and comfortable, determine hydration and nutrition and assess circulation (by feeling toe temperature). Diagnose by eye and by instinct. The experienced observer can

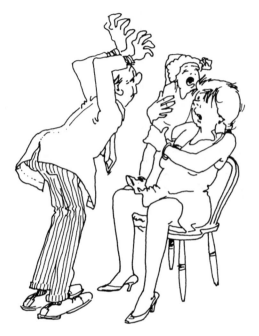

Fig. 4.13 The terrified toddler.

quickly decide whether the sleeping toddler is seriously ill or not.

Some toddlers defy proper examination despite stealth and patience. Try again when he may be in more benign humour. John Apley (a famous paediatrician) has said, 'It's my fault if a child cries'. We would not entirely agree. Toddlers have a very low threshold and tolerance for strange faces and stethoscopes. Occasionally you will meet the truly terrified toddler (a 'screamer') on whom examination is well nigh impossible. One may have to record failure:

Funduscopy – impossible
Blood pressure not recorded (crying)

and be prepared to try again later. Some 'tricks of the trade' are mentioned on pages 243–244.

Clinical conundrum : early sepsis

Sepsis needs to be considered in infants and young children with symptoms of fever, irritability, anorexia and lethargy. Such children may look pale and unwell, but localizing physical findings may be minimal or absent on examination. One needs to consider:

- bacteraemia/early septicaemia
- pyelonephritis (urinary tract infection)
- meningitis
- osteomyelitis.

By contrast, pneumonia is nearly always accompanied by physical signs – tachypnoea, grunting, flaring of alae nasi, and increased work of breathing.

Numbers to be recorded ('vital signs')

height
weight
head circumference
pulse (heart rate)
respiratory rate
blood pressure (where appropriate)
peak expiratory flow rate (where appropriate)
temperature

ILL acronym
Irritable
Lethargic
Low capillary refill

5 Systems examination

THE CHEST

The single most common reason for infants and toddlers to present to their family doctor is an acute respiratory tract infection, usually upper (see Ear, nose, mouth and throat). However, the good observer can often distinguish between infections involving the upper and/or lower respiratory tract (U/LRTI) by looking and listening carefully. All too often students are keen to get their hands and stethoscopes into play. Better to stand back and observe.

Observe the pattern of breathing, the work of breathing and the rate of breathing. Listen for an expiratory grunt. Note the type of cough. Does the infant display frothiness or flaring of the alae nasi? Does he have a wheeze? Can he cope with a feed? What is his colour like?

History

The history in respiratory tract infection consists of some combination or permutation of the symptoms of cough, wheeze, stridor, croup, poor feeding and fever. In more severe cases there may be rapid respiration, grunting, cyanosis, restlessness or even collapse.

It is very difficult to individually distinguish viral from bacterial infections. However, we have found 'Lightwood's law' to be of some value: this states that bacterial infections tend to localize – to one ear, to a tonsil, to a lobe of lung – whereas viral infections tend to spread. Measles is a good example of a spreading virus – red eyes, red ears, red throat, red skin and, if you could see it, red trachea. 'Toxicity' is difficult to describe clinically. Children with severe bacterial infections tend to be more 'toxic' – more sick, more still, more mottled.

It is also useful to try to distinguish upper from lower respiratory infections, remembering that URTI and LRTI can co-exist. One should attempt to correctly sequence from the onset of symptoms, as for example:

- cough for 4 days
- poor feeding for 2 days
- fever for 2 days
- wheeze for 1 day
- dyspnoea for 1 day.

It may be important to ask:

- Which came first, the cough or the wheeze?
- Is he getting progressively worse?
- Has he maintained a good colour?
- Can he manage a bottle or feed?

The four components of examination of the respiratory system are inspection, palpation, percussion and auscultation. Of these, inspection is surely the most valuable, especially in infants. By inspection we include listening as well as looking. We find ourselves frequently reminding students that the experienced paediatric ward sister can make an accurate stab at diagnosis from the door of the cubicle nursing an infant with an acute respiratory infection.

Palpation and percussion are not particularly useful exercises in acute LRTIs in infants and toddlers. The liver is frequently pushed down by a flattened diaphragm, the trachea is rarely displaced and demonstration of hepatic or cardiac dullness not particularly helpful. Lobar pneumonias demonstrable as dullness to percussion are infrequent in infancy. It must be emphasized that the above remarks are applicable only to infants. In childhood the traditional arts of percussion and palpation, as taught in 'adult' medicine, are important.

Inspection

Inspection will include comments on and recording of:

1. Colour.
2. How the child is coping: Is he comfortable? Is he noisy but managing? Is he in respiratory distress? Is he unstable, with very laboured breathing?
3. What is his position of comfort?
4. Respiratory rate – What is normal for a given age? (see Table 5.1)
5. Chest movement. Is it symmetrical? Is there splinting of one side of the chest?
6. Chest shape. Is the chest overblown or barrel shaped? Is there pectus excavatum (hollow chest), pectus carinatum (pigeon chest) or Harrison's sulcus?

Table 5.1 Normal respiratory rate (at rest)		
Age	Range of normal (respirations/min)	Rapid
Newborn	30–50	>60
Infant	20–30	>50
Toddler	20–30	>40
Child	15–20	>30

7. Pursing of lips in expiration?
8. Presence of frothiness, nasal flaring or grunting?
9. Type of respiratory movement. Normal respiration is a quiet in-out movement of the chest.

Come to terms: breathing

tachypnoea	= increased rate of respiration
dyspnoea	= laboured or difficult respiration
hyperpnoea (hyperventilation)	= increased depth of respiration
orthopnoea	= dyspnoea at rest

Defining tachypnoea (WHO criteria)

in infants <2 months	>60 breaths/min
in infants 2–12 months	>50 breaths/min
in children >12 months	>40 breaths/min

WHO, World Health Organization.

Come to terms: chest shapes

pectus carinatum = prominent sternum; pigeon chest
pectus excavatum = marked sternal depression
Harrison's sulcus = indrawing of lower chest with rib flaring (diaphragmatic tug)

10. Dyspnoea? This will be manifest by increased respiratory effort 'at rest'. Increased work of respiration is shown by suprasternal, intercostal and subcostal recession. Unilateral recession is sometimes seen in lobar pneumonia or with inhaled foreign body.

Increased rate and work of respiration are the most important signs of pneumonia in infants.

11. Is there finger clubbing? Clubbing of fingers and toes in children is usually secondary to cyanotic congenital heart disease or to chronic suppurative lung disease. If unsure about finger clubbing, look at the great toe. Clubbing may also be familial or associated with chronic diarrhoeal states. Clubbed fingers have a loss of the angle between skin and nail bed, increased convex curvature in both directions, may be beaked, and demonstrate transverse fluctuation.

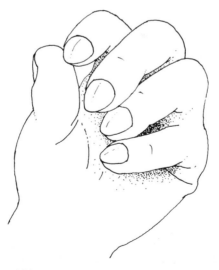

Fig. 5.1 Finger clubbing.

12. Presence of sputum: the expectoration of sputum is a relative rarity in young children, being mainly the province of children with chronic suppurative lung disease, for example cystic fibrosis. Even though a cough may correctly be called productive in infancy, sputum is not seen since it is swallowed. Evanson & Maunsell (1838) correctly stated: 'The young child almost always swallows any matter expectorated, and therefore this can scarcely become an object of diagnosis.' The swallowing of sputum is partly responsible for the vomiting which frequently follows a bout of coughing in childhood. Post-tussive vomiting is most typically seen in pertussis.

13. Traumatic petechiae may sometimes be seen on the eyelids, face and around the neck following a severe bout of coughing. They may also occur following prolonged crying or enforced restraint as for a lumbar puncture.

Palpation

Palpation should include a comment on symmetry and extent of chest expansion. Chest expansion should be about 3–5 cm in school age children.

The position of the trachea should be determined. Deviation of the trachea is infrequent in infants and toddlers.

Vocal fremitus can be assessed by palpation of the infant's chest when crying. Transmitted sounds may be palpated.

Percussion

Percussion should of course be performed gently, comparing sides. The percussion note in infants and toddlers tends to be more resonant than in adults. Detailed percussion in infants and toddlers may not be very rewarding. However, in the preschool child and schoolchild percussion should be carried out as in the adult.

Asthma at first sight?

Asthmatic children may have:

- jerky respiration (up-down chest movement rather than in-out movement)
- a tendency to raise their shoulders towards their ears on deep inspiration
- an overblown upper chest while the lower chest may have an early Harrison's sulcus.

Auscultation

The stethoscope

The stethoscope should preferably have a paediatric dia-phragm and bell; one sees many students today using the

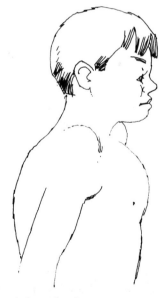

Fig. 5.2 Hyperinflated chest of asthma.

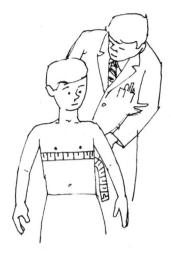

Fig. 5.3 Measuring maximal chest expansion.

diaphragm for all purposes. The bell is a much more useful sound-piece for infants, toddlers and children.

The bell is best

- The bell is smaller – the diaphragm of an adult stethoscope covers a large area of the chest of a neonate or infant.
- The bell is warmer – diaphragms can be very cold.
- The bell applies better to the chest.
- The bell allows less surface noise and is better attuned to receive low-pitched chest sounds. Indeed, the latter-day chest physician had no diaphragm on his stethoscope. Widespread use of the diaphragm for auscultating chests is undesirable and deplorable. The diaphragm is primarily designed for cardiac signs and sounds.

Auscultation implies use of the ear plus the stethoscope. Always listen carefully to the type of cough and attempt

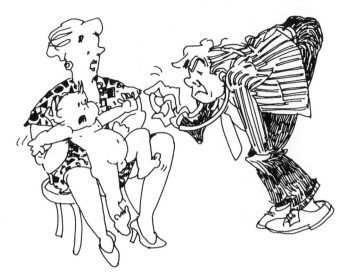

Fig. 5.4 Diaphragms can be cold, Doctor.

to describe it carefully. Listen for a grunt. An expiratory grunt is very suggestive of a pneumonic process. An audible wheeze, usually expiratory, is heard in a wide variety of childhood lower respiratory infections, from wheezy bronchitis to bronchiolitis to bronchopneumonia. An expiratory wheeze with prolonged expiratory phase is typical of bronchospasm associated with acute asthma.

It is important to remember that the stethoscope can be an unreliable instrument in the infant. One is occasionally struck by the finding of pneumonia on chest radiography in an infant whose chest seemed remarkably clear.

A few words on transmitted sounds. These are often heard in infants, especially frothy, mucousy infants, and can cause confusion for students. Transmitted sounds are sounds transmitted from the oropharynx to the chest, and are common in infants and toddlers. These noises arise from secretions in the upper respiratory tract, especially the oropharynx. Suction, coughing and physiotherapy may clear such sounds. They are rough, sometimes leathery sounds that are often mistaken by students for a pleural rub at first hearing.

The thin walls of the infant's chest allows easy conduction of sound from one side to another and gives the impression of increased intensity of breath sounds to the unfamiliar ear. Breath sounds in infancy have a broncho-vesicular character. In the preschool and schoolchild breath sounds assume the familiar vesicular quality heard in the adult.

One needs to develop the ability to listen between cries, to ignore surface movements and transmitted sounds and to compare intensity of breath sounds from side to side.

Pleural rub is an infrequent finding in preschool children. Ausculation of childrens' hearts or lungs through clothing is utterly unacceptable.

Adventitious sounds

Wheeze = rhonchus = continuous sound = dry sound.
Crackle = crepitation = discontinuous sound = wet sound.

Wheeze in infants is due to air movement through a narrowed airway, the narrowing of the tube being caused by:

- mucosal oedema
- excessive mucus
- bronchospasm.

Of these, bronchospasm is probably the least important. Several studies have failed to show any appreciable effects of bronchodilators on wheezy infants under 1 year of age. We can all see the 'runny nose' of rhinitis; consider the 'runny chest' as analogous. Wheeze can occur in a variety of chest infections, as shown below.

> **Wheeze-associated respiratory infections (WARI)**
>
> acute laryngotracheobronchitis
> acute bronchitis
> acute bronchiolitis
> acute bronchopneumonia

There is lack of uniformity and consistency in the terminology of acute bronchitis. We accept the terms 'wheezy bronchitis' and 'spasmodic bronchitis' as synonymous. 'Winter bronchitis' is not a helpful term. Most infants who wheeze in infancy wheeze infrequently and with infection. When wheeze is recurrent the correct term is usually 'asthma', or if you wish, 'asthmatic bronchitis'. There are, of course, other causes of recurrent wheeze including aspiration syndromes, foreign body, cystic fibrosis and tracheal compression.

A useful exercise in many systems, including the respiratory system, is to draw out one's findings in diagrammatic form. Some examples are shown in Figures 5.5 and 5.6.

Rhonchi (wheeze, dry sounds) and crepitations (crackles, rales, wet sounds) are no different in children than in adults and we will not describe them. However, it is wise to remember that rhonchi in infants are generated by air flow through a tube narrowed by oedema and mucus rather than being due to bronchospasm per se.

In approaching diagnosis in respiratory infection we find it useful to divide the respiratory tract into upper, middle and lower. One too often meets the lazy diagnosis 'URTI' or 'chest infection' in charts today. This represents clinical vagueness and uncertainty. One should attempt to be more specific. There are at least six URTIs and 'chest infections'. In a similar vein, the modern term 'pneumonitis' is equally imprecise.

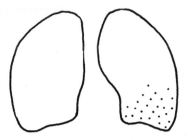

Fig. 5.5 Left basal crepitations.

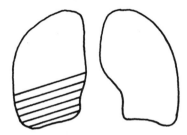

Fig. 5.6 Right middle and lower lobe consolidation.

Upper respiratory tract infection (URTI)		
rhinitis	otitis	sinusitis
tonsillitis	mastoiditis	pharyngitis

The term 'croup' has come to be a diagnosis. It is not. The word 'croup', from the Scottish word 'croak', describes the harsh, crowing, vibratory inspiratory stridor, usually accompanied by a barking cough and hoarseness. Croup has many causes, including infection, allergy and foreign body.

Middle respiratory tract infection (croup)

spasmodic laryngitis
laryngotracheobronchitis (LTB)
epiglottitis (supraglottitis)

Similarly, the diagnostic designation of 'chest infection' is not worthy of a medical student or doctor. 'Chest infection' is a layman's term. Again, there are many types of infection involving the lower respiratory tract.

Lower respiratory tract infection (LRTI)

tracheitis	pneumonia	bronchiolitis
bronchitis	bronchopneumonia	empyema

Although diagnosis in acute respiratory tract infection rests on a summation and interpretation of the findings, experience has taught us that certain signs in infancy are highly suspicious of certain conditions. Some examples are listed in Table 5.2.

Somebody has described grunting as a form of 'auto-PEEP': that is, automatic positive end-expiratory pressure.

Table 5.2 Signs highly indicative of underlying condition

Sign	Condition
Croup	Laryngitis, LTB
Wheeze	Wheezy bronchitis (Table 5.3)
Full chest, frothiness	Bronchiolitis (Table 5.4)
Flaring, grunting	Bronchopneumonia (Table 5.5)

Table 5.3 Wheezy bronchitis

Symptoms	Signs
Cough	Tachypnoea, recession
Wheeze	Audible wheeze
Low-grade fever	Bilateral rhonchi
Variable upset	

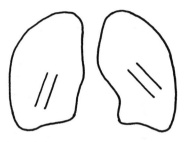

Fig. 5.7 Wheezy bronchitis.

Table 5.4 Bronchiolitis

Symptoms	Signs
Cough	Oral frothiness
Wheeze	Respiratory difficulty
Rapid breathing	Over-inflated chest
Poor feeding	Diffuse crepitations
	Bilateral rhonchi

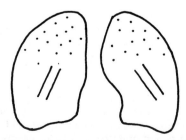

Fig. 5.8 Bronchiolitis.

Table 5.5 Bronchopneumonia	
Symptoms	Signs
Cough	Flaring of nasal alae
Wheeze	Grunting
Irritability	Respiratory difficulty
Fever	Unilateral or bilateral crepitations
Poor feeding	Occasional rhonchi

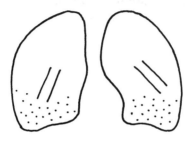

Fig. 5.9 Bronchopneumonia.

Occasional chest findings

1. *Pleuritic pain*: children with pneumonia do occasionally complain of sharp, severe pleuritic pain. Those old enough will point to the area. Younger children may 'splint' the affected side. In our experience a pleural rub is a rare finding in childhood, particularly in preschool children.
2. *Pneumothorax*: a small pneumothorax or pneumomediastinum may occasionally complicate acute asthma or a severe coughing spell in childhood (for example with pertussis). The pneumothorax is not usually clinically demonstrable; however, auscultation of a loud crunching noise synchronous with cardiac systole is characteristic.
3. *Subcutaneous emphysema* is sometimes seen in acute asthma. The cardinal clinical sign is a crackling feeling over the upper anterior chest, over the clavicles or in the neck.
4. Children with asthma sometimes complain of an itch in their throat.
5. *Tracheal pain* is a prominent feature of acute bacterial tracheitis.

Textbooks tend to try to classify and may at times over-simplify. Bronchiolitis and bronchopneumonia can in practice be difficult to distinguish, the balance being tipped one way or the other, perhaps, by chest radiograph or peripheral white cell count.

A compendium of coughs

Coughs may be dry or moist (productive). A productive cough results from an inflammatory or infective exudate on the bronchial mucosa. An intermittent or persistent dry cough may imply irritation of the upper respiratory tract or of the bronchial wall by a foreign body or extrinsic mass (glands). The appearance and amount of sputum should be assessed, remembering that children under 5 years swallow sputum. Clear mucoid sputum or tacky tenacious sputum is often indicative of asthma. Green, yellow, grey ('dirty') sputum usually indicates the presence of infection. Haemoptysis is now a rare phenomenon in children in developed countries, other than in children with advanced cystic fibrosis.

Listen to coughs and try to describe them. Below are listed some of the commoner varieties.

- Croupy cough: barking associated with stridor and hoarseness.
- Whooping cough: inspiratory gasp, prolonged distressing cough, ending in a whoop, followed by vomiting.
- 'Chesty' cough: moist, fruity, productive cough.

The type and timing of a cough (Table 5.6) can be important in deciding on the underlying respiratory problem.

Bacterial or viral illness?

Some simple clinical generalizations may assist in separating viral from bacterial aetiology bearing in mind that exceptions to rules always occur.

Table 5.6 Type and timing of cough

Cough	Suggests
Non-productive nocturnal	Postnasal drip, asthma
On exercise	Asthma
Paroxysmal	Pertussis, foreign body
During or after feed	Inhalation
Productive in morning	Cystic fibrosis, asthma
Bovine brassy	Tracheitis
Absent during sleep	Psychogenic

1. Viruses tend to spread to several sites – throats, ears, skin. A typical example is the diffuse redness of measles.
2. Bacteria tend to localize to one site – lobe of lung, single joint, abscess. However, bacteraemias and septicaemias certainly occur.
3. Bacteria tend to produce pus: for example, follicular tonsillitis. However, infectious mononucleosis produces a creamy tonsillar exudate.
4. Children tend to be more toxic with severe bacterial infections. Delirium, for example, is typically associated with pneumococcal pneumonia.

Suspect pneumococcal pneumonia

delirium
pleuritic pain
rusty sputum
herpes labialis (cold sore)

The following illnesses can be confidently diagnosed as almost certainly being viral:

- rhinitis
- pharyngitis
- laryngotracheobronchitis
- bronchiolitis
- wheezy bronchitis.

The infant/toddler with systemic viraemia looks miserable, has watery, puffy eyes, runny nose, usually a rash and often a harsh cough.

THE CARDIOVASCULAR SYSTEM

Congenital heart disorders (CHD), with an incidence of close to 1 per 100 neonates, are the second most common defects encountered. About half of congenital heart disorders may be detected in the neonatal period; the remaining will not present until later – hence the importance of routine examination at various ages. There are some 40 described varieties of CHD, of which only about 10 are frequent. For convenience we might classify them as follows:

Cyanotic CHD:	transposition of the great vessels
	Fallot's tetralogy
	pulmonary atresia
Potentially cyanotic CHD (left-right shunts):	atrial septal defect
	ventricular septal defect
	patent ductus arteriosus
Obstructive CHD:	coarctation of aorta
	pulmonary stenosis
	aortic stenosis.

The *symptoms* and *signs* suggesting congestive cardiac failure associated with congenital heart disease in infancy are:

- tachypnoea (respiratory rate > 50–60 breaths/min at rest)
- dyspnoea at rest or following a feed – inability to finish a feed due to dyspnoea is characteristic
- sweating – some refer to the circle of sweat on the sheet around the infant's head as the 'halo sign'
- unusual weight gain, greater than expected for caloric intake.

The weight gain signifies fluid retention

- tachycardia (heart rate >140–160 beats/min at rest)
- hepatomegaly
- gallop rhythm
- cyanosis, especially central – nursing the infant in 100% oxygen may help to distinguish cardiac from respiratory cyanosis.

Note: Pulmonary crepitations and oedema are relatively late signs of cardiac failure.

Temperature and heart/respiratory rate

1°C → increased heart rate: 10 beats/min
1°C → increased respiratory rate: 4 breaths/min

Approach to cardiovascular examination

Start at the periphery and work towards the heart. Look for cyanosis, clubbing, respiratory difficulty, anaemia or poly-cythaemia. Jugular venous pulse and pressure are difficult to appreciate in infancy due to the relative shortness of the neck.

We would agree with John Apley's approach to exami-nation of the heart: 'Use your eyes and hands before your ears. Leave the heart to last; and when you come to it leave auscultation to the last'.

The pulse

Pulses should be felt over the radial, brachial and femoral arteries. Preferably use finger pulps; if in difficulty use of thumbs is allowable, if not desirable. Femoral pulses, often difficult to palpate, must always be sought, otherwise coarc-tation of the aorta will be missed. If femoral pulses are thought to be diminished, look for evidence of radio-femoral delay – this can be hard to detect at rapid heart rates. Palpation of the dorsalis pedis pulse effectively excludes coarctation in infancy. Preauricular pulse is easily felt in sleeping infants.

Pulse volume

Is the pulse of normal, full or small volume? Appreciation of normal volume, with the finger pulp or tips, implies palpation of many pulses. Full volume pulses, due to a wide pulse pressure, are best appreciated at the radial pulse; easily palpable foot pulses in neonates and infants may be indicative of increased pulse pressure.

A thready, weak or small volume pulse is indicative of reduced pulse pressure. Most often it is felt in hypotension or impending shock in infants. Pulsus paradoxus is an appreciable change in pulse volume with respiration.

Pulse rate

Pulse rate is related to age and activity with variations brought on by distress, fever, excitement and exercise. The value of simple but careful observation of the pulse can be emphasized by the fact that the earliest signs of rheumatic fever are (a) a fixed tachycardia (no variation between sleep and awake pulse) and (b) loss of sinus arrhythmia.

The pulse rate will rise approximately 10 beats/min for every 1°C rise in temperature. The normal heart rate at rest is shown in Table 5.7.

Normal pulse variation

- *Sinus arrhythmia* – an increase in pulse rate on inspiration, with slowing on expiration. Very common in children.

Table 5.7 Normal heart rate at rest		
Age	Average rate	Upper limit of normal
0–6 months	140	160
6–12 months	130	150
1–2 years	110	130
2–6 years	100	120
6–10 years	95	110
10–14 years	85	100

- *Occasional ectopics* – need be of no concern.
- *Bradycardia* (pulse rate <60 beats/min) in fit children and adolescents, especially in good swimmers.
- *Slight tachycardia* with excitement due, for example, to clinic attendance or hospital admission.

Blood pressure

This is dealt with below. Postural hypotension is an infrequent finding in children. Appreciation of postural hypotension (a fall of 20 mmHg systolic blood pressure on adopting the upright posture) is an important sign of hypovolaemia.

Blood pressure should be routinely measured in infants and children with congenital heart disease. Indeed we suggest blood pressure measurement on all children admitted to hospital, on most attending outpatient clinics, and in all sick neonates and infants.

Colour

Central cyanosis is easily detected. Prolonged central cyanosis may result in plethoric appearance due to polycythaemia. Children with severe cyanosis sometimes adopt the squatting position after exercise – this increases peripheral resistance, increases pulmonary venous return and increases left-to-right shunting of blood.

Clubbing is dealt with on page 91.

Blood pressure (Tables 5.8 and 5.9)

The most obvious statement about children's blood pressure is that it is not taken. Not taken at all, not taken often enough, or not taken seriously. It is too often held that measurement of blood pressure in infants and children is difficult and time-consuming, and results are usually normal. Measurement of blood pressure in children merely requires patience, practice and a selection of cuffs from 3 cm to 13 cm wide.

Technique

Record blood pressure on right arm.
Child preferably seated or standing.

Table 5.8 Normal systolic blood pressure (BP)			
Age (years)	Systolic BP (mmHg)	Standard deviation	Upper limit of normal (+ 2SD)
1 (neonate)	60–70	10	90
1–4 (toddler)	90	10	110
6	100	10	120
8	105	10	125
10	110	10	130
12	115	10	135
14	120	10	140

Alternatively, systolic BP = 100 mmHg at age 6 years. BP rises by approximately 2.5 mm/year thereafter. (From Report of Task Force on blood pressure control in children. Paediatrics 1977; 59: 803.) Some 'rounding off' of standard deviation and other figures has been done for easier memorability. None of the figures quoted differs significantly from 'Task Force' values.

Table 5.9 Normal diastolic blood pressure (BP)

Age (years)	Diastolic BP (mmHg)	Standard deviation	Upper limit of normal (+ 2SD)
2	62	8	78
4	64	8	80
6	66	8	82
8	70	8	86
10	72	8	88
12	74	8	90
14	76	8	92

Or 60 + age in years = approximately mean diastolic. (From Report of Task Force on blood pressure control in children. Paediatrics 1977; 59: 803.)

Some minor 'rounding off' of standard deviation and other figures has been done for easier memorability.

Up to the age of 12 years there are no appreciable differences between boys' and girls' BP.

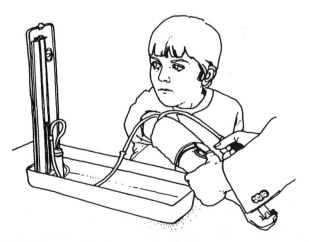

Fig. 5.10 Measuring blood pressure in children.

Child should be relaxed – pressures recorded during crying are unreliable.

Use the largest cuff width which comfortably fits the upper arm.

Ensure the inner bladder encircles the arm.

Doppler ultrasound recording for neonates and infants.

Standard auscultatory sphygmomanometry for older children.

Keep arm–heart–sphygmomanometer on same horizontal plane.

Diastolic pressure preferably recorded at point of muffling (phase 4). There is no clear point of muffling in about 5% of children. When this occurs, record phase 5 as the diastolic pressure.

If there is significant difference between phase 4 (muffling) and phase 5 (disappearance of sounds), record both points.

Suggested shorthand notation for blood pressure:

- ⚲ Standing
- ⚲ Sitting
- ∘–< Lying

Note the arm used and the cuff size.

Remember that anxiety plus faulty technique are probably the commonest explanations of elevated blood pressure in children. Single raised values are of no significance; they must be repeated several times. Blood pressures recorded on admission to hospital are notoriously unreliable. The combination of anxiety plus obesity in the child may also falsely elevate blood pressure. Getting the child to watch the mercury rise and fall can be helpfully distracting (Fig. 5.10).

In the newborn, especially if sick, Doppler ultrasonic methods or oscillometric methods provide the most accurate and reproducible measurements of blood pressure. The flush method is an unreliable measure of blood pressure.

In infancy, the standard auscultatory method can be used with patience and perseverance. By and large, toddlers do not like having blood pressure recorded, and there is a dearth of good data in this age group.

From age 5 years blood pressure is easily recorded in children, and some commentators are now suggesting that it be recorded annually – not necessarily to detect abnormality but to establish normality. A range of cuff widths – 7 cm, 9 cm, 11 cm and 13 cm – will be required. We use the simple rule that the largest cuff which fits comfortably around the arm should be applied. The child should be the recipient of any doubt concerning blood pressure recording.

Frequent errors in blood pressure measurement

failure to perform
cuffs that are too small
anxious, crying children
oscillations around systolic blood pressure – if you cannot hear phase 1
   or phase 5, deflate and start again
over-reliance on automated machines.

The heart

Having documented pulse rate, volume, blood pressure, colour, respiratory rate and effort, one may proceed towards the heart. Here the classical skills of inspection, palpation, percussion and auscultation apply. We shall only refer to findings applicable to children.

Inspection

Here one is seeking two major things:

- a precordial bulge
- visible ventricular impulse.

A precordial bulge will cause the sternum and ribs to bow forwards, giving the chest an overblown appearance. The right ventricular impulse may be visible under the xiphisternum. The left ventricular impulse (or apex beat) is frequently visible in thin children, in children with hyperdynamic circulation (due to fever or excitement) and in children with true left ventricular enlargement.

Palpation

Palpation implies localization of the apex beat, a search for right or left ventricular enlargement, and an appreciation of palpable sounds or murmurs. A palpable murmur is referred to as a *thrill*.

Right ventricular enlargement is best sought with one's fingertips placed between 2nd–3rd–4th ribs along the left sternal edge. Some people prefer to use the side of their hand when assessing the right ventricle. The abnormal palpation in right ventricular hypertrophy is called a tap or a lift. A slight right ventricular tap may be felt through the chest wall of thin children; it is a normal finding. The apex beat is found in the 4th intercostal space along the midclavicular (or nipple) line in infants and toddlers. It may be difficult to localize in plump, healthy infants and toddlers. If you cannot locate the apex beat, think of dextrocardia or a pericardial effusion (both rare phenomena).

In schoolchildren the apex beat is in the 4th–5th left intercostal space in the midclavicular line. Left ventricular hypertrophy can result in a diffuse, forceful and displaced apex beat. The feeling is described as a *heave*.

Palpation of a thrill is always significant. A thrill in the suprasternal notch may suggest coarctation or aortic stenosis. A palpable heart sound usually implies accentuation of that sound (usually pulmonary second sound). Palpation may reveal whether the heart is active or hyperdynamic.

Percussion

We do not find percussion of the heart particularly helpful. However, you may be asked to demonstrate cardiac percussion in an examination. The technique is as for an adult.

Auscultation

Auscultation, as stated earlier, should always be left to last, remembering then the old adage – 'sounds first, murmurs second'. Insofar as students are concerned the majority of murmurs are systolic until proved otherwise. If you can appreciate diastolic murmurs at the fast heart rates of infancy, you are well tuned into auscultation. We do not propose to reiterate the routine of cardiac auscultation, which is the same at all ages.

When listening:

- try to ensure the child is not crying
- use both diaphragm and bell (preferably paediatric sizes)
- listen with the child in lying and sitting positions
- note any variation with respiration.

Sounds first. The first sound is best heard at the apex with the bell and the second at the base with the diaphragm. In infancy, the first sound may be louder than the second. A soft first sound is an early sign of carditis. The first sound may be normally split.

The second sound is usually split in children, this split being physiological and widening on inspiration. A third heart sound may be a normal finding in some children.

Murmurs. Insofar as students are concerned paediatric murmurs pose two problems:

- hearing them at all
- distinguishing between a significant and an innocent murmur.

113

When listening for murmurs try to wipe out all extraneous noise and listen between the first and second sounds *very carefully*, using both diaphragm and bell in all cardiac areas. It is usual to grade murmurs 1–6 in an arbitrary fashion for recording purposes. We propose the simple system given in the box.

Murmur mnemonic
grade 1: barely audible, innocent
grade 2: soft, variable, innocent usually
grade 3: easy to hear, intermediate, no thrill
grade 4: loud, audible to anybody, thrill
grade 5: sounds like a train, very significant, thrill
grade 6: scarcely requires a stethoscope, thrill

Murmurs of grades 4–6 are always significant. Grades 1–2 are usually innocent, and grade 3 is intermediate. The length of the murmur is important, pansystolic implying significance, midsystolic suggesting innocence.

Innocent murmurs (also known as physiological, ejection, or flow murmurs) are very common in childhood (being heard in up to 50% of children). Their distinguishing features are displayed below.

Innocent murmurs: usual features
midsystolic
soft in intensity (grades 1–3)
localized
poorly conducted
musical or vibratory in character
variable with position and respiration
not associated with other signs of heart disease

Significant murmurs: usual features

pansystolic
conducted all over precordium
soft to loud (grades 4–6) in intensity
associated with a thrill
accompanied by other signs, e.g. ventricular enlargement
any diastolic

One innocent murmur which may cause difficulty is the *venous hum*. This is a low-pitched, continuous, rumbling murmur, best heard under the right clavicle. It is usually louder when sitting up, diminishes on lying, and may be abolished by obliterative pressure over the internal jugular vein.

The first hurdle for the student is to distinguish significant murmurs from innocent murmurs. Clearly all murmurs must be properly described – systolic, diastolic, loudness, duration, point of maximal intensity, conduction, etc. Diastolic murmurs are relatively infrequent in children and so require extraordinary auscultatory care if they are to be heard. If the student can determine that the murmur is significant, the next step will be to determine its origin. This will require consideration of colour, pulses, ventricular impulses, heart sounds and the characteristics of the murmur. At undergraduate level, examiners are usually content with elicitation and elucidation of murmurs. If pressed towards a diagnosis, the following points may help:

- cyanosis + murmur   usually Fallot's tetralogy
- cyanosis + murmur + operation   possibly Fallot's tetralogy or transposition of great arteries
- pink + loud systolic murmur   probably ventricular septal defect (the single commonest form of CHD)

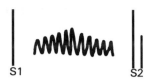

Fig. 5.11 A cardiac murmur.

- pink + murmur + impalpable femorals
- continuous low-pitched murmur

probably coarctation of aorta

possibly patent ductus arteriosus

It is good practice to draw a diagram of the features of a cardiac murmur (Fig. 5.11).

THE ABDOMEN

In this section we propose to discuss the routine examination of the abdomen, including the genitalia and rectum. We will not refer to palpation or auscultation of the 'acute surgical abdomen'. First a few words on vomiting.

Vomiting

Vomiting requires definition and in terms of amount, remember that mothers and nurses tend to overestimate volume of vomitus. What is its frequency and timing? What does it contain – undigested milk, blood, food, bile? Is it forceful or effortless? Try to distinguish projectile vomiting from regurgitant, apparently effortless vomiting. Separate small 'spits' from true vomits. All babies vomit occasionally. Is the vomiting related to feeds? Are feeding volumes appropriate? Is he hungry after he vomits? The statement 'He's still hungry despite the vomiting' is very characteristic of pyloric stenosis. Does the vomiting bother him? Does the vomiting bother his mother? What has she done about it?

Inspection

The abdomen in toddlers and children is usually protuberant in the upright posture. Even experienced physicians have difficulty distinguishing a normal 'pot-belly' from a pathological one. Abdominal protrusion is often related to exaggerated lordosis in the upright position.

Respiration is normally abdominal in type up to schoolgoing age. Small umbilical hernias are a frequent finding. Slight separation (divarication) of the rectus muscles is normal. Distended veins may be noted. Visible loops of bowel are sometimes noted in malnourished infants.

Abdominal fat in growth hormone deficient children resembles 'cellulite' in adults.

Epigastric hernias are infrequent. By contrast inguinal hernias are common, especially in the male infants. Intra-abdominal masses are occasionally visible. Wilms' tumours can come to medical attention when parents note the swelling on bathing their child. Draw in and label any operative scars you inspect.

Abdominal distension is often gaseous. Simple percussion can help to distinguish between solid, cystic and gaseous distension. Abdominal distension could be:

- fat
- fluid
- faeces
- flatus
- visceromegaly
- muscle hypotonia
- exaggerated lordosis.

117

Palpation

It is of prime importance to have the infant and child relaxed when trying to palpate the abdomen. This will require patience, skill and distraction techniques. Hands must be warm. Try to avoid making the child cry! You may occasionally have to palpate the abdomen with the infant crawling. Some toddlers will allow you to palpate their abdomen while standing, but object vociferously once you lie them down.

The purpose of abdominal palpation is to:

- seek the presence of normal abdominal structures.
- detect enlargement of abdominal organs.
- seek abnormal masses or fluid.

Feeling the spleen

The spleen is to be found in the left upper abdominal quadrant and is normally palpable 1–2 cm below the left costal margin in infancy. It is soft and can be tipped on inspiration.

The enlarged spleen moves on respiration, is dull to percussion, has a notch and one cannot get above it. Don't poke for spleens. Lay your right hand gently on the abdomen and allow the spleen to come to meet it, with your left hand below. Splenic size should be recorded in centimetres below the costal margin. Very large spleens can be missed, if one fails to begin palpation below the umbilicus and work slowly upwards. The splenic notch is occasionally visible. With chronic enlargement the spleen will usually become firmer. It is rarely tender. The spleen may enlarge medially towards the umbilicus or downwards toward the left iliac fossa. Splenic enlargement tends to be directly downwards in infancy.

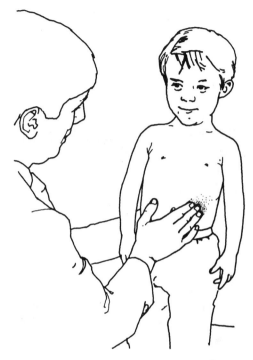

Fig. 5.12 Palpating the abdomen of the toddler standing on a couch.

Palpating the liver

The liver is a relatively busier and larger organ in infants. A liver 1–2 cm below the right costal margin is considered normal up to the age of 2–3 years. The liver when enlarged is easily palpable in infants and children. Its edge is soft and it moves down with respiration.

When palpating for the liver don't poke as this will provoke tightening of the abdominal muscles. Approach from the right iliac fossa (RIF) with the tips of the fingers

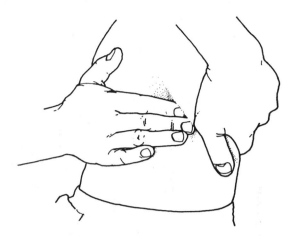

Fig. 5.13 Palpating the spleen.

or the side of the index finger, lay one's fingers gently on the abdomen and allow the child's respiratory movement to bring the liver to meet your fingers.

Measure liver breadth in centimetres, not fingers. It can be useful to percuss out liver dullness and to express total liver size in centimetres, rather than its level below the costal margin. However, determining the upper border may not be easy. Liver span is 6–12 cm in children aged 6–12 years. A normal-sized liver may be pushed down by a flattened diaphragm, as in bronchiolitis.

The liver breadth below the costal margin is a very useful indicator of congestive cardiac failure in infants. Indeed enlargement of the liver can be the earliest sign of incipient cardiac failure.

We have not found the scratch test to be particularly helpful in determining liver size. Palpation and percussion should suffice.

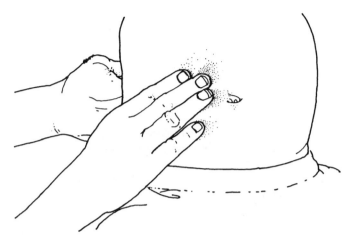

Fig. 5.14 Palpating the liver.

There are many causes of hepatomegaly in children, from storage diseases to tumours. Liver tenderness is sometimes seen in acute hepatitis.

In summary, the liver is characterized by the following:

- a palpable edge in the right hypochondrium
- movement with respiration
- dullness to percussion
- inability to get above the swelling.

Palpable nodules and audible bruits over the liver are distinctly unusual in paediatrics. Liver smallness (or atrophy) is almost impossible to clinically designate in children, since inability to palpate a liver is not in itself abnormal.

The kidneys

The kidneys are not easily palpable in infants and children, despite the claims by some authors. Indeed we would say to the inexperienced student – if you can palpate the kidneys they are probably enlarged.

In the hypotonic newborn the kidneys (especially the lower pole) should be palpable and ballotable. Kidneys move on respiration, have a smooth outline, and one can get above them. Kidneys are best palpated bimanually; we have not been impressed by the technique of using the thumbs on anterior approach. The normal fetal lobulation of the newborn kidney is not clinically appreciable.

Enlargement of the kidney in the newborn may be bilateral or unilateral. If unilateral, consider congenital mesonephroma/nephroblastoma (Wilms'), multicystic dysplasia, hydronephrosis, renal vein thrombosis (where the kidney is strikingly firm). If bilateral, renal enlargement may indicate polycystic disease, bilateral obstructive uropathy (secondary to urethral valves) or congenital nephrotic syndrome.

Bladder

The bladder can be palpated in the neonate and infant (since it is an abdominal organ) and is easily percussible when full. A very full bladder may sometimes be visible.

Genital examination

Students need to be aware that children are modest, shy and are taught to be reticent regarding genital inspection by strangers. It is therefore very important for students to introduce themselves, explain who they are, what they are doing and why they are doing it.

Inspection and examination of the genitalia is a routine part of examination of infants, toddlers and schoolchildren. More is learnt by inspection than by palpation.

Genital examination should *always* be performed in the presence of the mother or a nurse.

Under no circumstances should unsupervised examination of the vagina be performed in young girls. The normal vaginal appearances can be learned from videos. Inspection of the perineum is part of the examination of girls. It is not, however, necessary to separate the labia or do any form of internal examination. If the labia need to be separated, this is best done by the mother.

In boys, inspection of the penis and testes is part of the routine examination. In the male one is looking for normality (or deviation therefrom) of the penis, scrotum and testes. Students need to check that the penis is of normal size, that the meatus is properly positioned and that the testes are descended. Many 'undescended testes' are found on re-examination to represent retractile testes; the over-hasty approach of cold hands has induced a brisk cremasteric reflex. Indeed any self-respecting testis will 'run for cover' if approached threateningly in this fashion. Don't attack the testes! Occasionally retraction of the foreskin may be necessary to detect phimosis, etc. The examination of male external genitalia can be often satisfactorily performed by inspection only.

Is the urethral orifice at the normal position on the tips of the glans? If not is there epispadias (dorsal opening) or hypospadias (ventral opening)? Hypospadias may be glandular (common), penile (rare) or perineal (very rare) (see p. 60).

Male genitalia

Enlargement of the penis occurs in certain endocrine and neurological conditions. Note that in congenital adrenal hyperplasia the penis is large, but testicular volume is normal. The commonest explanation of a small penis is a normal penis buried in fat. True micropenis (where there may be little palpable other than penile skin and urethra) is rare. Normal penile lengths and circumferences have been published.

Inspection of the scrotum should reveal normal rugosity and visible testes. In toddlers and boys, testes are best examined in the standing position. The next choice is lying flat on the couch, and the final attempt is made with the child in a squatting position. The squatting position helps to abolish the cremasteric reflex and is most valuable in those cases of retractile testes (Fig. 5.16).

A small, flat, underdeveloped scrotum may signify true maldescent. If uncertain about undescended testes always repeat the examination. Undescended testes are a common finding in preterm baby boys.

Knowledge of normal testicular volume is an attribute not obtained by most practitioners; all that is required is an

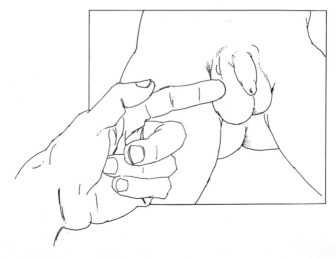

Fig. 5.15 Cremasteric reflex.

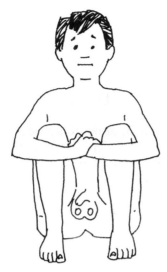

Fig. 5.16 Squatting for examination of testes.

appreciation of approximate normality. Prader (of Zurich) has produced an orchidometer (or 'testicular rosary') giving a range of testicular volumes. Awareness of testicular volume may be important, for example, in assessing children with leukaemia (the testes may be a site of relapse), or in following a surgically corrected torsion of the testis (is the testis growing normally?).

Enlargement of the scrotum may be due to an enlarged testis, a hydrocele (transilluminable) or an inguinal hernia. Hydroceles are common in neonates.

Female genitalia

The vulva is usually inspected in girls. Adhesions of the labial mucosa are not infrequent. Vaginal palpation is not usually performed unless there are clear-cut clinical indications, such as suspected foreign body, suspected sexual abuse, vaginal discharge.

The clitoris is prominent in preterm baby girls. A bloody postnatal vaginal discharge ('newborn period') is an occasional normal event. The uterus and ovaries are not normally palpable in infants and children.

Come to terms: abdomen	
atresia	= closed lumen
omphalocele (exomphalos)	= midline hernia containing abdominal contents, sac covers
gastroschisis	= paramedian hernia, no sac
urachus	= embryological connection from bladder to umbilicus

Examining for ascites

Ascites in the newborn may be:

- a transudate, as in hydrops, heart failure
- an exudate, in peritonitis
- biliary (rupture of common bile duct)
- urinary (spontaneous or traumatic rupture of the bladder)
- chylous (rupture of lymphatic duct).

Of the above, only a transudate is in any way common. Ascites is also seen in chronic liver disease and is a fairly frequent accompaniment of the nephrotic syndrome in childhood.

The ability to demonstrate ascites is frequently sought by examiners, and is therefore an important clinical skill to acquire correctly.

Gross ascites:

- may be obvious on inspection
- the abdomen is distended
- the umbilicus is everted
- there are obvious pressure marks on the skin
- the flanks are full
- the skin looks oedematous
- the vulva or scrotum are full.

A 'fluid thrill' is an unreliable sign, and can easily be elicited (incorrectly) in very obese children. More reliable by far is the sign of 'shifting dullness'. In looking for dullness one should percuss from resonant (above) to dullness (below). If there is definite dullness in the flank, the child should be rolled onto one side, and a change to resonant percussion note sought – 'shifting dullness'. One must be careful not to percuss over the iliac crest in determining flank dullness. The distribution of ascitic dullness is 'horseshoe shaped'. The child should be allowed to lie on his side for 30–60 seconds before checking for dullness. The child with ascites

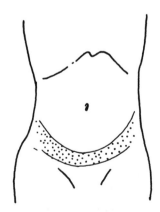

Fig. 5.17 Distribution of ascitic fluid.

may have a 'jelly belly': that is, a feeling of free mobile fluid in the abdomen.

Putting your finger in the rectum

Rectal examination is not routine in children. Always explain to children before you do it. Tell him you hate doing it, but have to. Always use lubrication. Relax the child as best you can. Rectal examination is most often done in acute abdomens, chronic constipation and rectal bleeding. Use the little finger for little children (neonates and infants) and index finger for older children. Lie the child on his side with legs drawn up. Approach the rectum from the inferior, always taking the opportunity to inspect the perianal area prior to inserting one's finger. One occasionally may see threadworms, skin tags or protruding polyps. Haemorrhoids are rare in children. On spreading the buttocks apart, anal fissure may become apparent. Anal fissures (fissure-in-ano) are most often seen at 6 and 12 o'clock and may be accompanied by sentinel tags (Fig. 5.19).

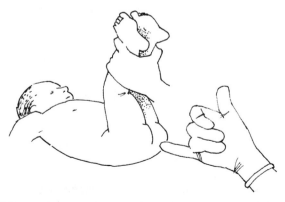

Fig. 5.18 Rectal examination.

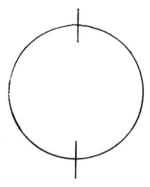

Fig. 5.19 Anal fissures.

On insertion of one's finger anal tone can be easily assessed. A tight anus resisting one's finger is suggestive of anal stenosis. A loose patulous anus usually indicates a lower spinal lesion such as myelomeningocele or diastematomyelia.

In examining the rectum one is looking primarily for:

- masses (faeces, polyps, teratomas)
- local abdominal tenderness
- blood or other staining on the examining glove.

There are mixed surgical opinions on the value of rectal examination in the clinical situation of 'acute abdomen ?appendicitis' in children. We would suggest that it is a useful procedure as one may detect tenderness (in a retrocaecal appendix) and occasionally an appendix mass.

Rectal prolapse and rectal polyps are infrequent findings in paediatrics. Although children put foreign bodies in all sorts of orifices, rectal foreign bodies are unusual. Mothers occasionally bring in roundworms and tapeworms which have been passed per rectum; these should always be kept for proper identification.

Inspection of the underwear and perianal region is important in the child with faecal staining and soiling. Rectal examination may be valuable in distinguishing between constipation with overflow incontinence ('spurious diarrhoea') where the rectum is full of hard faeces, and behavioural soiling where one finds soft faeces in the rectum.

The anus should always be inspected in the newborn to ensure that it is perforate; imperforate anus is easily missed, especially in baby girls who may pass meconium through a vaginal fistula. Hirschsprung's disease is among the causes of neonatal intestinal obstruction – the explosive release of flatus is said to be characteristic.

The 'anal wink' or anocutaneous reflex, which is contraction of the anus on stroking the perianal region, should be sought in infants with spina bifida.

Child sexual abuse

The recognition of the frequency of child sexual abuse has exposed doctors' unfamiliarity with normal genital and anal appearances and variations in children. We believe that it is beyond the remit of this text to cover child sexual abuse in detail, and would suggest that normal and abnormal findings will best be learned from slide photographs and videos. Nonetheless, it is important that students and doctors appreciate normal introital and hymenal variations in girls. The normal anal appearance is very variable. The effects of constipation need to be distinguished from penetrative sexual abuse. Reflex anal dilatation (widening of anus on separation of the buttocks) is not necessarily abnormal or pathological.

Other abdominal findings

1. *Faecal masses* can be felt in the central and left lower abdominal quadrants. Sometimes referred to as 'faecal rocks'

they are mobile, indentable and non-tender. Remember that immobile children, particularly with severe cerebral palsy, frequently become constipated.

2. *Trichobezoar* (a hair ball) is a rare finding in the stomach of disturbed children.

3. *Tumours*: large tumour masses include nephroblastoma, neuroblastoma, cystic teratoma, hepatoblastoma, mesenteric cysts. These are most often found in infants and toddlers.

4. *Ovaries* are not usually palpable in girls. Enlarged palpable ovaries are associated with ovarian cysts, teratomas and tumours.

5. *Adrenal glands* are never palpable, even though relatively large in the newborn. Enlargement of the adrenal is a feature of tumours – usually phaeochromocytoma and neuroblastoma.

EXAMINING THE GLANDS

Children are frequently brought to doctors because of cervical lymph nodes whose apparent persistent enlargement can be a source of concern to parents. Neck glands may be readily visible in thin children. Needless to remark, an unspoken fear of leukaemia may initiate the consultation. Most often these 'swollen glands' are normal, reflect recent infections, and need not cause worry. Small, pea-sized, discrete, non-tender, shotty glands are a normal finding in the cervical and inguinal chains in preschool children. Inguinal glands are occasionally palpable in newborn infants.

Enlarged unilateral axillary glands are often felt after neonatal bacille Calmette-Guérin (BCG) vaccination. They are usually due to local inflammation/infection at the injection site. Rarely one sees tuberculous axillary lymphadenitis after BCG.

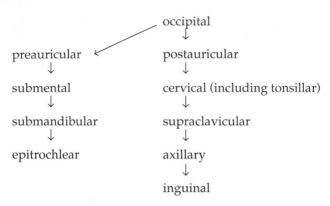

Fig. 5.20 Lymph nodes: top-to-toe palpation.

Examination of the lymphoreticular system is an integral part of the examination of the child. One may either systematically go over areas where lymph nodes may be felt, or seek them during examination of individual body systems. We suggest that lymph nodes are best palpated in a methodical, systematic fashion from 'top to toe' – it takes but a short time.

Neck glands should be examined from both behind and in front of the child. Site, size, consistency, tenderness, mobility and attachments of nodes should be carefully recorded. The diameter of single enlarged nodes should be noted. If many lymph glands are enlarged, one must always look for splenomegaly and hepatomegaly.

Persistent enlargement of cervical lymph nodes usually reflects acute tonsillitis. Although acute tonsillitis subsides rapidly, the draining nodes take much longer to do so. Children with atopic eczema frequently have enlarged regional lymph nodes. Generalized lymph node enlargement should initiate a search for acute infection, inflammation or neoplastic process (see box).

Lymph node enlargement

Cervical lymphadenopathy:
tonsillitis, pharyngitis, sinusitis
chronic gingivostomatitis
'glandular fever' (infectious mononucleosis/cytomegalovirus)
tuberculosis (uncommon in developed countries).

Generalized lymphadenopathy:
acute exanthemata
'glandular fever'
systemic juvenile chronic arthritis (Still's disease)
acute lymphatic leukaemia
drug reaction
mucocutaneous lymph node syndrome (Kawasaki's syndrome).

CLINICAL EVALUATION OF THE IMMUNE SYSTEM

Nowadays the immune system is usually evaluated via a series of laboratory parameters, including serum immunoglobulins, white cell function and lymphocyte subsets. Useful clinical examination can, however, be gleaned from physical examination.

Clinical evaluation of immune system

Are the tonsils present?
Are the lymph glands palpable?
Has the BCG vaccine taken? (This is a test of lymphocyte transformation.)
Any pustular skin infections?
Any allergic rashes?

EAR, NOSE, MOUTH AND THROAT

The ear

The ear is low-set when the helix (top of the pinna) meets the cranium at a level below that of a horizontal plane with

133

the corner of palpebral fissure. Pain on pulling the pinna suggests a boil in the external canal. Many mothers suggest that children with otitis media 'pull their ears' or that the pinna is red in middle ear infections.

Abnormalities of the pinna are seen in many syndromes, from Treacher Collins to Down's syndrome. It has been said, but not substantiated, that abnormalities of the external ear are associated with kidney abnormalities; the association is a weak one. Cosmetic abnormalities such as protruding ears ('bat ears') are common. Large ears have been described in fragile X syndrome.

Examining the ear drums

It must be said that otoscopy is frequently poorly performed by students – they rush at the child, fail to instruct the mother properly, use too small a speculum and sometimes hurt the child.

The mother should gently but firmly hold the child against her chest, one hand over the forehead, the other hand around the chest grasping the child's hands. The legs may be held between the mother's thighs if necessary.

In the infant the pinna should be pulled downwards since the canal is directed upwards. In the older child pull the ear up to direct the drum towards the visualizing otoscope. Not infrequently wax will obscure one's view. Should it be removed? Certainly not by the inexpert student.

Always use the largest speculum you expect to fit. We prefer the penhold grip as this allows the otoscope to move readily with any movement of the child. Inspect the canal on the way in.

If the child is fearful of otoscopy, demonstrate it first on the mother. Do not push the otoscope in more than 0.5 cm in infants or 1 cm in older children. One may see otitis externa or a furuncle (exquisitely painful) in the canal. One

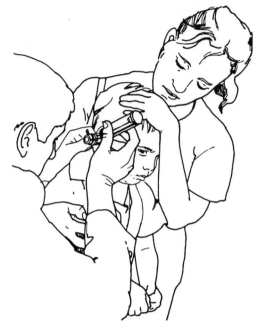

Fig. 5.21 Examining the ear.

occasionally comes across an unexpected foreign body, such as a bead.

The normal appearance of the drum is greyish-white and translucent with a clear light reflex. The most common abnormality to detect is redness, which, if accompanied by bulging, implies middle ear infection.

Pinkness or redness of the drum is readily determined. Remember that crying may suffuse the drum and give the false impression of 'inflammation'. We have been impressed by the difficulty in locating perforations when pus is exuding from the canal.

135

A dull, retracted or full drum with loss of light reflex is indicative of serous otitis media (commonly known as 'glue ear'). This condition, which has several causes, is due to obstruction of eustachian tube drainage.

Mastoiditis is now a very infrequent condition. Acute mastoiditis can be associated with protrusion of the pinna, and with redness and swelling over the mastoid. More likely today a postauricular swelling or tenderness would be caused by lymph node inflammation. Preauricular sinuses or pits can be seen in front of the ear; they are congenital but sometimes may become infected.

Treat the ear with restraint and respect and it will repay you with an appreciation of how redness, retraction and perforation really appear.

The nose

Respiration in the newborn is usually nasal; nasal obstruction can result in considerable respiratory difficulty, even apnoea. Air movement through each nostril can be detected by feeling flow with one's fingertip, by listening with the stethoscope, or by noting condensation on a mirror held over the anterior nares. If in doubt, in the newborn, nasal patency can be established by the passage of a catheter. Unilateral or bilateral choanal atresia is a rare finding.

A flat nasal bridge is usually normal. However, it is a notable feature of Down's syndrome.

The nose is a common receptacle for foreign bodies (beads, etc.) which may result in unilateral purulent discharge. The nose may be examined using the auriscope – gently. A boggy nasal mucosa may suggest allergy. Nasal polyps suggest asthma or cystic fibrosis. A chronic, mucopurulent nasal discharge through the winter is a frequent finding in cold climates.

A common complaint concerns the child with persistent nasal discharge ('runny nose'). The discharge may be clear (as in viral or allergic rhinitis) or purulent (suggesting sinusitis or adenoidal obstruction). Bloody nasal discharge (epistaxis) often results from nose picking. Spontaneous epistaxis usually originates from a minor vascular malformation of the nasal mucosa (Little's area). Parents (understandably) exaggerate blood loss in epistaxis.

The mouth

The oral cavity is hostile and often unexplored territory to innocent practitioners, paediatric and general alike: mouths that won't open, jaws clamped on a prising spatula, teeth ready to snap on probing fingers, a fleeting glimpse at tonsils and quivering uvula. Infants and small children do not like to have their mouths and throats examined. Hence this examination should be left until just about last. Some will open as wide as a yawning alligator on the promise that a spatula will not be used. Others have to be coaxed into cooperation. Sometimes pressing a finger into each cheek will force open the mouth. When necessary the child could be appropriately restrained (Fig. 5.22).

The tonsils

Proper inspection of the tonsils requires a good light source, a well-opened mouth and a speedy observer.

The tonsils can be surprisingly difficult to visualize in neonates and infants as the tongue seems always to ride up. It is remarkably and embarrassingly easy to miss a cleft of the soft palate in the newborn. One occasionally comes across a bifid uvula, which may be associated with a submucous cleft soft palate.

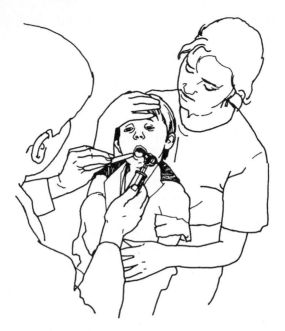

Fig. 5.22 Examining the mouth and throat.

One has a few fleeting moments to observe redness, exudate, or secretions in the oropharynx. The classic streptococcal tonsillitis produces a unilateral or bilateral follicular exudate. A creamy, confluent exudate is typical of infectious mononucleosis; other noteworthy features of this illness are palatal petechiae and a swollen uvula. Some texts state that infectious mononucleosis does not occur in young children; this has not been our experience. Diphtheria, though now rare, must not be forgotten. It causes a severe lymphadenitis, 'bull neck', a greyish membrane and notable toxicity. It needs to be stated that gonococcal tonsillitis may have to be considered in atypical or unresponsive infections in adolescents.

While examining the tonsils the student should also look at the oropharynx for evidence of pharyngitis, exudate or a postnasal drip. Postnasal drip may be elicited by asking the child to say 'aah' at length.

Tonsillar size is not important unless extreme. By extremely large tonsils we mean tonsils that meet in the midline (sometimes referred to as 'kissing tonsils'). Repeatedly infected tonsils may have a pitted appearance.

The tongue

A large protruding tongue is a feature of congenital hypothyroidism. Macroglossia may also be caused by a local lymphatic or vascular anomaly. The tongue may appear inappropriately large for a small mouth as in Down's syndrome. A geographical tongue is a tongue with irregular red lines and pale areas. It is of no particular significance.

A white-coated tongue is usually attributable to a recent milk feed. Monilial infection (thrush) is manifest by a patchy white exudate which cannot easily be removed by a spatula. Herpetic stomatitis affects the tongue, mucosa and buccal border. It is vascular, friable, bleeds to touch, and is associated with marked drooling.

Buccal mucosa

Thrush appears as serpiginous white patches on the mucosa. Koplik's spots are like a grain of salt with a red rim; they are found in the buccal gutter during measles prodrome. Inflammation of the parotid duct usually implies acute viral parotitis (mumps). Recurrent suppurative parotitis (with or without stone) is a rarity in childhood.

The teeth

Dentists have a modicum of medicine. Doctors have a minimal knowledge of dentistry, which is virtually absent from most medical curricula. Particularly in early childhood, the doctor has a unique opportunity to practise some preventive dentistry. Even a brief look into the child's oral cavity and a scan of teeth and gums is a useful exercise. Below are some spin-offs of dental examination:

1. Dental caries is prevalent still, especially in the less well-off segments of society. Caries of the upper incisors is sometimes called 'nursing bottle caries'.
2. Early detection of maleruption, malocclusion and malalignment.
3. Dental staining may be of diagnostic significance. Dental enamel hypoplasia has been described as a sequela of neonatal hypocalcaemia. Brown or yellow staining (which

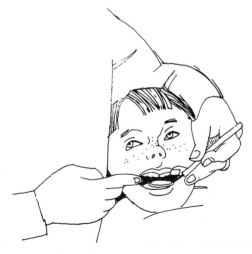

Fig. 5.23 Inspecting the teeth.

fluoresces under Wood's light) is a side-effect of tetracycline consumption in pregnancy and early childhood. Black staining of the teeth sometimes follows iron ingestion.

4. Flattened teeth are seen in normal and handicapped children who grind their teeth (bruxism).
5. Absence of teeth is a feature of ectodermal dysplasia.
6. Gingivitis is frequently associated with caries. Gingival hypertrophy, with or without gingivitis, occurs in children consuming phenytoin and ciclosporin long term.

Come to terms: oral cavity

ranula	= cyst on anterior floor of mouth
quinsy	= peritonsillar abscess
glossoptosis	= backward displacement of tongue
micrognathia	= small chin

SKIN, HAIR AND NAILS

In this section we mention some normal skin variations, some clinical clues to be found in skin, hair and nails, and propose that the secret of success in skin conditions lies in inspection, palpation and description. We shall not refer to acute infectious exanthemata.

Skin

Skin colour. Discussion of racial variations in skin colours is beyond our remit. Students will be aware of increasing cross racial relationships allowing for all sorts of pigmentary variations.

Mongolian blue spots are black or navy areas over sacrum, buttocks and sometimes shins of infants of Middle Eastern,

African and Asian parents. Pigmentation of the scrotum may be an associated finding.

Absence of skin pigmentation occurs in albinism, which is easily missed at birth as the pink lens may not be noted and skin pigment is light in most infants. Skin pigmentation increases through infancy.

Freckles (multiple small pigmented spots) are fairly common, especially in fair-skinned people.

Café-au-lait spots are pigmented patches more than 1.5 cm in diameter. When greater than six in number they may suggest neurofibromatosis; axillary freckles are characteristic of this conditions.

Small bruises on the forehead are a normal finding in toddlers, who have recently acquired the skill of walking. Similar small bruises (as many as 20) are a frequent finding on the knees and shins of preschool and schoolchildren. The characteristic sites and appearance of bruises suggestive of non-accidental injury are described elsewhere (see Chapter 11).

Carotenaemia (yellow discolouration of the skin) has been described in infants and children consuming excessive amounts of carrots and mandarin oranges.

Vitiligo is an area of depigmented skin, and may be seen in tuberous sclerosis and autoimmune conditions.

Come to terms: hair/skin	
hirsutism	= excessive hairiness; synonym 'hypertrichosis'
hyperhidrosis	= excessive sweatiness
lentigines	= brownish pigmented spots on skin
vitiligo	= depigmented patches

Sclerema is an erythematous thickening and hardening of the skin associated with hypothermia or vascular stasis. Local sclerema is usually confined to hands and feet. Generalized sclerema indicates a serious systemic disorder.

Oedema. Generalized oedema of the skin is a normal finding in preterm infants. Hydropic conditions of the newborn are accompanied by generalized pitting oedema. Dependent oedema is unusual in the newborn but may occur in the propped infant in congestive cardiac failure.

Lymphoedema (non-pitting) is classically found in the lower limbs in Milroy's syndrome (congenital lymphoedema) and in the XO neonate (Turner's syndrome).

Erythema nodosum is a red, painful raised swelling on the tibial surface (shin). The lesions may vary in size and number. It is associated with streptococcal infection, drugs, tuberculosis, inflammatory bowel disease and sarcoidosis.

Hair

Hair colour, thickness and distribution are racial attributes. Soft downy hair (lanugo) is found in preterm infants. Bushy head hair at birth is a normal variant, but may suggest congenital hypothyroidism. Bushy eyebrows are a feature of mucopolysaccharidoses and of de Lange syndrome. Long eyelashes are a normal (sought after) attribute in girls; they also occur in children with chronic debilitating disorders.

Prominent dark hair on forearms, nape of neck, and back is a normal variant. White flecks in the scalp hair are a feature of Waardenburg's syndrome. Kinky hair is described in the rare Menkes' syndrome. Lank 'lifeless' hair is sometimes noticed in coeliac disease.

Absent or short occipital hair may be a feature of infants who are either delayed or deprived; it reflects too much time spent in the supine position. Children with Down's syndrome typically have straight hair. Total absence of hair is seen in ectodermal dysplasia (a rare condition), and as a side-effect of cytotoxic drugs.

Local absence of hair in a child may reflect either alopecia or trichillomania (hair pulling). In alopecia the area may be totally bald; in trichillomania short hair roots are usually present.

Nits (pediculosis capitis) are a common finding nowadays. They are adherent to hair shafts, difficult to displace and need to be distinguished from dandruff. A paediatric predecessor of ours used to refer to head lice as 'mechanized dandruff'.

Excessive hair (hypertrichosis, hirsutism) may be a side-effect of several drugs, including phenytoin, diazoxide, minoxidil, ciclosporin and corticosteroids.

Nails

Nails are often long in the post-term (postmature) neonate. Absence of nails is a feature of ectodermal dysplasia. Peripheral cyanosis of nail beds (acrocyanosis) is a normal newborn variant.

Spoon-shaped nails (koilonychia) are occasionally a normal variant; they may be associated with anaemia. White lines across the nails (leuconychia) can be seen with chronic hypo-albuminaemic states, such as nephrotic syndrome and liver disorders. Small white spots on the nails do not indicate calcium deficiency.

Pitting of the nails is described in fungal diseases and in psoriasis. Nail biting is a frequent finding in children, stressed and unstressed.

The secret of success in skins

The secret of success in dermatology is to describe what you see. Stand back, look carefully at the rash and apply descriptive terms to its colour, appearance, distribution, feel, etc. Too many students take one look, and jump at a diagnosis like a salmon at flies. It is better by far to use one's power of description and palpation.

Today's students can be inhibited by a lack of even a smattering of Latin or Greek, which certainly helps in understanding skins. The student who knows some Latin would not call the uniform circular lesions of psoriasis 'erythema multiforme'. Included below is a glossary of some classic terms in an effort to overcome confusion.

We suggest that once you have seen the following rashes you immediately and carefully describe them:

- psoriasis
- tinea corporis (ringworm)
- erythema nodosum
- anaphylactoid purpura
- molluscum contagiosum.

It is worth assembling a clinical differential of red rashes, purple (purpuric) rashes, vesicular rashes and bullous eruptions.

Examination of skin rashes

inspection
palpation
description
distribution

Glossary of dermatological terminology	
erythema	= redness
erythema multiforme	= redness of many shapes
erythema marginatum	= red raised margin
erythema annulare	= red, circular
atopic eczema	= literally means 'out of place boiling over', 'atopy' from *topos* (Greek for place) eczein = to boil over
centrifugal	= fleeing from the centre
centripetal	= seeking the centre
morbilliform	= measles-like
varicelliform	= chickenpox-like
ichthyosis	= dry, scaling skin. From *ichthus* (Greek for fish)

Describe a rash as though you were attempting to describe it to a blind person – site, size, colour, shape, distribution, feel. Is it a macule, papule or vesicle? Is it itchy? Is it wet or dry? Is it centrifugal or centripetal? Is it raised or flat? What does it feel like?

Come to terms: rashes	
macule	= flat lesion
papule	= raised lesion
vesicle	= fluid-filled lesion
bulla	= large vesicle
pustule	= vesicle containing pus

Eczema (atopic dermatitis) is the commonest chronic rash in childhood. Eczema is a good example of applying description in order to come to a conclusion. The skin in eczema may be:

- erythematous (red)
- dry
- papular (palpably raised)
- scaling (ichthyotic)

- excoriated (scratched)
- thickened (lichenified)
- weeping (? infected).

Insofar as children are concerned, four irritations of eczema are:

- itching
- ichthyosis
- infection
- image (of self).

Palpation of the rash is most important and frequently not performed. Few rashes in paediatrics are painful. Measurement of lesions and clinical photography are very useful for recording purposes.

Desquamating rashes. Desquamation means shedding or peeling of skin. Desquamation is not common, but can be diagnostically alerting. Among those children's rashes which desquamate are:

- Kawasaki's disease: desquamation around nail edges, on hands and feet and in the nappy area is typical
- scarlet fever
- severe measles
- staphylococcal scalded skin syndrome.

Petechiae or purpura? Purpuric rashes are important in paediatrics. There is some confusion and overlap between these terms. We have always understood petechiae to be fine, non-blanching, non-palpable purple spots usually around 1 mm in diameter. Purpura are also purple, non-blanching spots of 2 mm or more. Purpura may be palpable. Purpura has many causes; however, a rapidly spreading purpuric rash in infancy is suggestive of septicaemia. The rapidity of onset, spread, distribution and association with bruising are relevant clinical factors. The degree of sickness (or wellness!) is important. 'Wet' purpura (on mucosal surfaces) used to be considered more serious than 'dry' purpura (on skin). Common causes of purpura include:

- acute meningococcal septicaemia. The appearance of spreading purple spots in an acutely unwell infant or child. Parents in the UK have been taught on television to do the glass test – the spots fail to blanch when a glass is rolled over them.
- coagulopathy, most commonly idiopathic thrombocytopenic purpura. The child is usually well and the purpuric spots are accompanied by ecchymoses and bruises.
- vasculopathy, most commonly Henoch–Schönlein purpura. The purpuric rash is most prominent on buttocks, backs of legs and arms.

There are many causes of purpura, and the clinical discussion is very much related to the child's age, the differential being very different in the newborn than in the adolescent.

It is important to remember that skin, teeth, hair and nails are all ectodermal structures and should be seen as a continuum, particularly when dealing with congenital abnormalities of some part of the system as in ectodermal dysplasia. The state of the hair and skin, in particular, can contribute to a clinical assessment of a child's state of nutrition.

Nappy rashes = ACES
ammonia
Candida
eczema
seborrhoea

Napkin area rashes:

- seborrhoeic dermatitis (scalp, neck and axilla also involved)
- ammoniacal irritant dermatitis (skinfold flexures usually spared)
- *Candida* (thrush) dermatitis (satellite lesions are characteristic)
- eczema (typical lesions elsewhere)
- acrodermatitis enteropathica (a rare condition associated with zinc deficiency)
- erosive or ulcerated napkin dermatitis is a severe form of irritant ammoniacal dermatitis.

Napkin area rashes are very common and need to be seen and, if possible, clinically separated as outlined above. The four major causes are seborrhoea, ammonia, *Candida* and eczema.

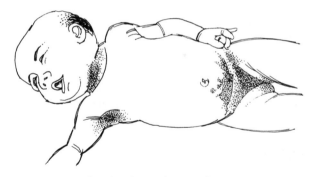

Fig. 5.24 Nappy rash (seborrhoeic dermatitis).

Chilblains (perniosis) are sometimes seen in children living in cold houses in cold climates. They are noted on the fingers, toes and occasionally the ears; they are inflammatory blisters, which may ulcerate. Keratosis pilaris, or dry bumpy skin on the arms and legs is common and often familial.

Come to terms: skin infections

cellulitis	= redness, heat, swelling due to superficial skin infection in various sites
impetigo	= blistered, crusted, brown skin lesions on face and limbs
scalded skin	= erythema, burn-like areas, may be widespread

Intertrigo may be observed in overweight infants and children. This is a wet, red eruption in furrows between opposed skin surfaces of the groin, axilla and sometimes neck.

In summary, examination of any rash must include:

- inspection
- palpation
- good description.

Come to terms: 'derm'

dermatoglyphics	= study of fingerprint and hand crease patterns
dermatographia	= skin writing. white line with red margins following scratching of skin
dermoid	= teratoma of skin structures
Dermatophagoides pteronyssinus	= house dust mite

NEUROLOGICAL EXAMINATION

We do not propose to exhaustively deal with the neurological system, but rather to present some points about the neurological system and its examination that are *different* in infants, toddlers and preschool children. Neurological examination at these ages cannot always be performed in an organized fashion.

By contrast a 'classic' full neurological examination can be carried out on a cooperative schoolchild. Its tricks and techniques are fully described in your basic text on clinical methods so we will not elaborate further. The neurological examination of the neonate is described in Chapter 4. Intrinsic to an understanding of the infant's neurological system is that maturation of the central nervous system (CNS) is manifest by a loss of primitive reflexes with a corresponding gain in positive skills. Developmental examination, including speech, hearing, gross and fine movement, is presented in Chapter 8.

The neurological approach combines:

1. Careful history of birth, perinatal events, developmental sequence, maternal worries, etc.
2. Observation of the infant's activity, symmetry and of the toddler's movement, play and socialization.
3. Expedient examination of tone, power, coordination, reflexes and sensation. Sensation can be especially difficult to ascertain in infancy.

History

One will need to enquire about movement in utero. Although maternal instincts about normal intrauterine movement may be fallible, in retrospect they may be alerting. Reduced fetal movement may be significant.

Perinatal events are important. Low Apgar scores (<5) at 1 and 5 minutes, though not in themselves prognostically valuable, may contribute to concern.

How did the baby suck? And move? Did he pass his neonatal neurological examination?

Tell me about his development. Was a normal pattern followed? When did he first smile with meaning? When did he sit unsupported, etc.? The modern mother may well have filled these developmental milestones in her baby's book or diary. If so, ask to look at it.

If a mother presents her infant with a possible developmental or neurological problem remember our primary:

- she's usually right
- her worries often commenced well before attending doctors
- her instincts are sharper than your observations.

Some alerting statements made by mothers

'He was an unusually good baby' (this may mean he cried or moved very little, but merely slept and fed).
'He was always different from the others.'
'He was okay till 9 months of age then he seemed to stop.'
'He seems to have gone backwards.'

Infants with perinatal insults tend to be abnormal in their behaviour from the beginning. Babies with neurodegenerative disorders, for example, may develop normally for a period and then stop, or indeed, regress.

Neurologists, above all specialists, are obsessive in their demand for a good history. When did the problem begin? What was the child like before that? What exactly happened? What has been the sequence of events since then? Giving a history of a convulsion to a neurologist as an intern is akin to being cross-examined in court by a querulous senior counsel. So learn the art before you qualify. Be confident, be complete and choose your words carefully. In other words, take a good history, or risk being 'hammered'.

Examination techniques

We plan merely to highlight some skills and certain signs particular to paediatrics. For detailed description of neurological examination refer to your text of clinical signs.

Tendon reflexes

The fingertip is sometimes used to elicit knee jerks in neonates; this is acceptable practice. After the newborn period we recommend the use of a small reflex hammer. When striking a tendon with the hammer, be a swinger not a stabber – in other words allow the hammer to have a free flowing stroke. The knee jerk is best tapped with the hammer held in a pengrip and parallel to the leg.

The use of the side of the stethoscope's diaphragm to elicit tendon reflexes is sloppy practice and not recommended.

Deep tendon reflexes may be arbitrarily graded for record purposes as follows:

0 = absent
1+ = weak response
2+ = normal response
3+ = exaggerated response
4+ = very brisk response

Exaggerated responses are characteristic of upper motor neurone (pyramidal) lesions, reduced reflexes occur with muscle weakness, and absent reflexes suggest a peripheral neuropathy (lower motor neurone).

Funduscopy

In infants and toddlers, funduscopy requires the patience of Job and a fair amount of skill. Funduscopy can at times be akin to seeking a passenger in a train rushing by. Do your best. Don't be depressed if you fail – we all do (see p. 188 for more detailed discussion).

Neonate

We will only briefly mention the newborn, whose neuro-logical examination is detailed in Chapter 4. Observe the posture adopted by newborn babies and infants. Observe limb movements and in particular whether symmetrical or not. Note the normal flexed position of the well infant. See the 'frog position' of the floppy infant. Look for neck extension in infants with 'cerebral irritation' or with severe meningism. Look for spontaneous movement and for abnormal movements.

Normal newborn findings:

- tremulousness
- mass responses
- extensor plantar response
- unsustained ankle clonus.
- Babinski response may be upgoing (extensor) to the age of 8 months.

Infant

How does the infant handle? This is an important observation. Does he resent handling (as, for example, infants with meningism)? Is he floppy – does he tend to slip through your hands in upright suspension? Is he stiff – does he tend to move 'in one piece'? Is muscle tone decreased?

Cranial nerve examination

Full formal cranial nerve examination can be difficult in infants and toddlers. However, observation of everyday activities such as smiling, crying, sucking, looking, ruminating and chewing can be very instructive. Examination of the 1st cranial nerve is almost impossible in preschool children; fortunately it seems rarely involved in neurological disorders. Table 5.10 lists activities requiring normal cranial nerve function for perfect performance.

The commonest cranial nerve problems in infants include squint (paralytic or concomitant) and facial nerve palsies

Table 5.10 Activities requiring normal cranial nerve function		
Activity	Cranial nerves used	Comment
Smell	1	Impossible
Visual acuity	2	Can he see?
Eye movement	3	Up, medially, down, in
Eye movement	4	Down and out
Chewing	5	Or rooting
Eye movement	6	Lateral
Crying, smiling	7	Facial expressions
Hearing	8	Startle reflex, formal testing
Sucking	5, 7, 9	Serious if absent
Swallowing	9, 10, 11	Coordinated?
Phonation	9	Or test gag reflex
Phonation	10	Observe palatal
Head turning	11	movement
Tongue protrusion	12	

(congenital or acquired). Poor or absent sucking in a term infant is a serious neurological sign. Failure of appearance of a social smile at 6 weeks warrants worried observation. Mothers are intimately tuned into their infants and usually acutely aware of social responses such as looking, hearing, smiling and cooing. The mother may often better elicit these responses than you can, but do try and do learn. Please remember that infants and toddlers respond best to friendly, smiling human faces in preference to lights, pens, toys or other inanimate objects.

At the end of the neurological examination it will be helpful to arrive at a broad general conclusion as follows:

1. Definitely normal in all respects.
2. Probably normal but shows a few minor discrepancies. Check again.

3. Probably abnormal. Definite deviations from normal, such as absence of social smile, weak suck, or reduced movement. Repeat examination.
4. Definitely abnormal. Definite findings such as absence of visual fixation, persistent primitive reflexes, altered tone (usually floppy), etc.

Neurological and developmental examinations are integrally interrelated and require lots of skill and practice. Students should confine themselves to the extremes – demonstration of normality and detection of major abnormality. The subtleties in between will accrue with postgraduate time and practice.

We believe that sensory examination of infants and toddlers is too subtle and too subjective for undergraduate students and will not discuss it further. Pain is easy to elicit but we would suggest that our primary premise – first do no harm – takes precedence. Fortunately, most neurological insults in infants and toddlers involve the motor system rather than the sensory system. Absence of sensation can be demonstrated in the flaccid lower limb paraplegia associated with myelomeningocele and in ascending polyneuritis (Guillain–Barré syndrome).

Disappearance of primitive reflexes with appearance of positive skills is part of the developmental sequence (Table 5.11). Persistence of primitive reflexes is neurologically sinister.

Table 5.11 Primitive reflexes: appearance and disappearance		
Reflex	Appearance	Disappearance
Stepping	Newborn	2 months
Moro	Birth	3–5 months
Palmar grasp	Birth	2 months
Plantar grasp	Birth	8–10 months
Asymmetric tonic neck	Newborn	1–6 months

Feeling the fontanelle

If the eye is the window of the soul, the fontanelle is a window on the infant's brain.

The tension of the anterior fontanelle is an important sign in deciding whether or not an infant has raised the intracranial pressure and in determining the presence and degree of dehydration. The fontanelle must preferably be palpated (gently!) when the infant is quiet or sitting upright. Fullness and elevation of the fontanelle over the surrounding skull is evidence of increased intracranial pressure. The usual causes of this will be meningitis or hydrocephalus. No comment should be made if the infant is crying.

A systolic bruit is frequently audible over the anterior fontanelle in the presence of meningitis. This usually disappears in 2–3 days.

Delayed closure (beyond 18 months) of the anterior fontanelle

Delayed closure (beyond 18 months) of the anterior fontanelle is associated with:
  normal variation
  hydrocephalus
  Down's syndrome
  hypothyroidism
  bone disorders
  some syndromes
  arteriovenous malformation.

A rapidly enlarging head may be a cause of concern. Serial measurements of head circumference are important. If a large head is accompanied by a full fontanelle and spread sutures, raised intracranial pressure is the likely cause.

Some causes of large head

familial macrocephaly (measure parents' heads)
hydrocephalus
space-occupying lesion
storage diseases
bone disorders
Sotos' syndrome

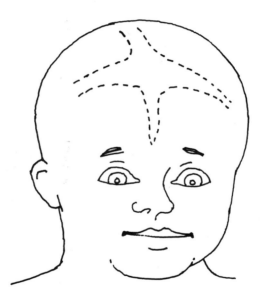

Fig. 5.25 Signs of hydrocephalus.

Head growth is a reflection of brain growth. However, except at the extremes, head size is not related to intelligence. When the head is small (*below third centile*) it is microcephalic.

Some causes of microcephaly
normal variation
perinatal asphyxia
intrauterine infection (TORCH)
chromosomal disorders
familial
dysmorphic syndrome
severe metabolic disorder

Enlarging heads can be sometimes halted; poorly growing heads, unfortunately, usually cannot be helped.

Eliciting neck stiffness

Meningism or neck stiffness is a very important sign to elicit correctly. The student needs to be gentle, always to look for active resistance to flexion before passive resistance, and to be aware of voluntary resistance exhibited by that *enfant terrible*, the fretful toddler. It is important to state at the outset that neck stiffness, unless severe and obvious, is an unreliable sign in the neonate and infant.

First, observe the infant's position of comfort. The well-relaxed child sleeps in a position of cuddled flexion. The ill infant may extend. The infant with severe meningeal irritation may adopt the position of *opisthotonos* or hyperextension of the neck and trunk.

Ask the toddler to follow a light. Ask the child to flex his chin onto his chest. Ask him to kiss his knee. In the sitting position ask him to look at the roof. If he can do all of these readily, neck stiffness is likely to be absent, or if present, minimal.

Then, while supporting his occiput, gently flex his neck, feeling for resistance to movement. In severe meningism the child will lift up 'like a board'. Lesser degrees of meningism may cause him to wince or cry on flexion. Always note

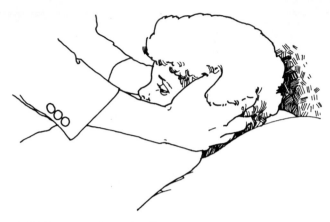

Fig. 5.26 Examining for neck stiffness.

carefully the facial expression when looking for meningism. Eliciting neck stiffness with the child sitting up with knees extended is another sensitive manoeuvre.

Neck retraction (or extension) arch is a more reliable sign of meningism than neck stiffness in infants.

Kernig's sign (resistance to straight leg raising)

This can be elicited in children and has the same significance as in adults. Kernig's sign is, however, unreliable under the age of 3 years. Kernig's sign is performed by flexing the hip and knee to a right angle (Fig. 5.27a) and then slowly extending the leg (Fig. 5.27b). A positive sign exists when there is pain and limitation of movement. While doing this manoeuvre it is useful to feel for tightness of the hamstring. The child may additionally demonstrate Brudzinski's sign by reciprocally flexing the contralateral knee in order to take the stretch off his lower spine.

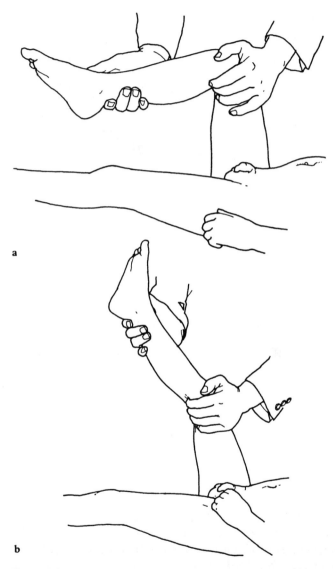

a

b

Fig. 5.27 Kernig's sign.

Meningism

Genuine meningism is likely to be associated with a shrill, high-pitched cry. The infant may be drowsy and irritable, may refuse feeds, and may wish to be left alone. Meningism does not always imply meningitis. It must be recognized that meningism may be associated with upper respiratory and other infections.

Some causes of meningism
meningitis, encephalitis
acute otitis media
severe tonsillitis
cervical lymphadenitis
pneumonia
retropharyngeal abscess

Toddlers

In mobile children more information about tone, power, coordination and movement is learned by the amateur neurologist through informal observation than by formal examination. So to assess motor progress, you will need to observe:

- walking
- running
- jumping   } gross motor skills
- kicking
- smacking
- climbing

- scribbling
- transferring   } fine motor skills
- picking up objects
- building blocks

You can practise on your nephews, nieces, or relations' children in the appropriate 1½–4-year-old age group. Children of this age are most willing performers who love to show off their prowess. Again, students need not concern themselves with the multiplicity and subtlety of variations but rather concentrate on knowing the normal and major deviations therefrom.

Skills achieved in all of these areas will be related to chronological and developmental age. The speed and dexterity with which the above motor skills are performed can be very informative. Be prepared to get onto the floor and observe *play*. Play is the all-consuming interest of inquisitive toddlers and preschool children. Our neurologist colleague informs us that she does much of her neurological examination at floor level. A period in the ward or hospital playroom will be well repaid. There you can notice constructiveness, concentration, conversation (children often speak to themselves when playing), coordination and curiosity. Mentally handicapped children may demonstrate short attention span, poor construction abilities, lack of concentration, absence of interest in other children or surroundings. Beneath the apparent chaos of the playroom, important business is being conducted.

At the bed or cot side a few bricks, pieces of Lego, or simple toys are invaluable. The combination of good maternal history, observation of manual dexterity and interest in toys may help you construct the beginnings of a neurological template.

At all ages it is important to observe:

- alertness (bright eyes, bright smile, bright face)
- activity
- social adaptation.

Note the toddler's *gait*, hand or foot preference (if determined) and in particular look for symmetry of movement.

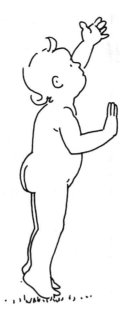

Fig. 5.28 Toddler standing on tiptoes.

Children with a hemiplegia tend not to want to use the hand on the affected side. Hemiplegia may delay the onset of walking; he drags the leg or limps. All gaits are unsteady for a while after acquisition of walking. Persisting unsteadiness, frequent falls and dropping of objects may suggest ataxia. Observation of play is imperative in determining coordination.

It is worth observing the gait of any child with a suspected neurological disorder. Children usually acquire the skill of independent walking between 10 and 18 months. The initial gait is unsteady and broad based; confidence and coordination are rapidly gained. Failure to walk independently by 18 months warrants an explanation (familial, obesity, bottom-shuffler?) and an examination to establish normality or determine the cause.

Certain *characteristic gaits* are worth noting and if possible videorecording:

1. Gait of muscular dystrophy is of a waddling nature, the hips being thrown from side to side.
2. Ataxic gait – usually wide based, unsteady and poorly coordinated.
3. Hemiplegic gait – tendency to drag and to circumduct the leg with extended foot, which scrapes the ground.
4. Lower limb weakness results in the foot being dragged and a slapping gait.
5. Toe-walking gait is not in itself abnormal and has been noted in infants born prematurely.
6. Possible causes of a limping gait are mentioned on pages 175–176. Remember that a late or missed congenital dislocation of the hip may not be apparent until the child walks.

Schoolchild (5+ years)

The cooperative schoolchild will usually allow you to carry out a complete formal neurological examination as appropriate. This is described in your text on clinical methods so we will not duplicate here. One will always have to make allowance for the child's confidence, cooperation and comprehension of what is required of him. The examiner will need to be patient, expedient and to be prepared to try again. Testing of children's sensation is not often required but when performed needs clear explanation to the child of the answers being sought (children are very obliging creatures and may give false answers for fear of disappointing you!).

In the schoolchild the following are the best tests of coordination:

- one leg stance
- hopping
- walking on tiptoes
- walking on heels.

The child aged 5 years or more who can hop is well coordinated. In our country little girls will often demonstrate their dexterity by dancing a simple jig or reel. In these circumstances, formal neurological tests such as straight line walking or running the heel along the leg, are stupid and superfluous.

In addition you may wish to observe the child writing, kicking a ball, tying his shoelace, clapping, catching a ball, buttoning his shirt. By the age of 5 years hand dominance is determined – most children are predominantly right-handed, right-footed and right-eyed.

The neurological examination is not complete without a clinical comment on:

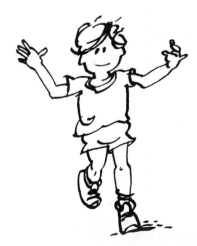

Fig. 5.29 One leg stance.

- vision
- speech
- hearing
- intelligence.

Come to terms: odd movements

chorea	= coarse, involuntary, purposeless movements
athetosis	= slow, writhing, incoordinate movements
tic	= repeated bizarre movements; habit spasms
tremor	= constant small movements
fasciculation	= random contractions of groups of muscle fibres
myoclonus	= sudden, single, shock-like contraction of muscles

---

Determination of tone

Tone implies resistance to passive movement and its assessment is related to age. In the newborn and infant, tone is best assessed by neck traction, by ventral and upright suspension, and passive movement of limb joints. Tone may be normal, reduced (hypotonic or floppy), or increased (hypertonic, spastic). The infant (post neonatal) who 'slips' through your hands in upright suspension is hypotonic. Hypotonia may be caused by muscle weakness or wasting (as in malnutrition, myopathies, cerebellar lesions and neuropathies). Wrists and ankle joints may be unduly floppy and muscles may feel flabby. Shaking of wrists and ankle joints is a useful index of tone in infants.

The characteristics of spasticity are increased tone of the muscles and exaggerated deep tendon reflexes. One has to work harder to flex and extend the joints involved. Rigidity may be of the 'lead-pipe' variety (the same throughout the range of movement), 'clasp-knife' (stiff initially, but gives), or 'cogwheel type' (jerky throughout).

A selection of CNS signs

1. *Cracked pot note* is the hollow, cracking note one obtains on percussing the skull in the presence of raised intracranial pressure and closed fontanellae. The examiner's ear is applied directly to the head and the skull percussed with one finger. In older children with space-occupying lesions and spread sutures a 'hollow note' may be elicited. The sound is quite different from the solid note of the sound skull. The sideroom technique of skull transillumination has been rendered superfluous by the advent of cranial ultrasound.
2. *Setting sun sign* is when the sclera is visible above the iris. It is seen in hydrocephalus with raised intracranial pressure. It is also seen in normal 'pop-eyed' infants.
3. *Head tilt* is an interesting and important sign. It may be evidence of torticollis and is seen in children with strabismus and ptosis. Rarely it has been described as an early sign of an occipital tumour.
4. *Doll's eye reflex* is where the eyes move in the opposite direction to that of the head.

Cerebral palsy

Definition: a disorder of movement and posture presenting in infancy and characterized by one or a combination of hypotonia, spasticity, ataxia, involuntary movements.

The common types of cerebral palsy are:

- hemiplegia
- quadriplegia – spastic
- diplegia
- ataxia
- dyskinesis – choreoathetosis, dystonia.

Hemiplegia (commonest type)

The upper limb is more involved than the lower limb. There is marked thumb adduction, fisting and increased pronator tone. Contractures may occur and limb growth may be retarded.

Quadriplegia

In this situation all four limbs are involved, particularly the upper. The predominant sign is hypertonia, demonstrable at the wrists and elbows, and also in the ankles, knees and hips.

Diplegia

The lower limbs are more severely involved with a symmetrical distribution. Clinical presentation coincides with development of extension in the lower trunk and hips. Typically the infant drags himself around the floor with flexed arms and extended legs. Extensor spasticity at the hips and knees results in the classic signs of extension and scissoring of lower limbs.

Orthopaedic deformities may result from the altered tone, including:

- kyphosis of the thoracic spine
- lordosis of the lumbar spine
- dislocation of the hips
- equino varus or valgus feet.

Ataxia

- Diplegia (as described above)
- Cerebellar involvement
- Initial hypotonia

- Intention tremor
- Stamping gait.

Dyskinesis

This implies irregular and involuntary movements of some or all groups of muscles. These movements may be continuous or be present only when the limb is deliberately moved. The signs of dyskinesis include hypotonia, slow and purposeless movements, involvement of distal parts of limbs, and accentuated voluntary movements.

Disabilities associated with cerebral palsy

- Mental handicap (IQ < 70) in 75%
- Visual – squint, refractive errors
- Hearing – partial deafness
- Speech – disorders of sensation, perception and language development
- Epilepsy
- Emotional problems.

The purpose of physical and neurological examination is to determine:

- the type of cerebral palsy
- the severity and distribution of the problem
- the nature and extent of associated mental and physical handicap.

MUSCULO-SKELETAL SYSTEM

In this section we have arbitrarily lumped together the limbs, muscles, bones and joints, with a few words on congenital malformations. A lot of interesting paediatric case material is to be found on the orthopaedic ward. We propose to highlight a few points in a chronological fashion – newborn, toddler and schoolchild.

A thorough examination is from head to toe. Most students are thorough in their systematic questioning and systems examination. Nonetheless the untrained eye can easily miss little things, which may be relevant – polydactyly, for example, or 2nd–3rd toe partial syndactyly (a common finding), or 5th finger clinodactyly. We have seen schoolchildren with Poland's syndrome (absence of the pectoralis major muscle and/or nipple) whose parents have failed to notice this apparently obvious deformity. Scoliosis is easily missed at any age unless one specifically looks for it.

Observe the infant or child in his preferred position. If mobile, watch how he moves around. Does he creep, crawl, bottom-shuffle? Observe the gait. Can he run? Note coordination, dexterity and symmetry of movement. Can he hop on one foot (a good test of coordination as well as muscular strength)? Can he jump? How does he get up from the sitting position? Has he a limp, waddle or other abnormal gait? Are the limbs symmetrical and of equal length? Parents will frequently seek medical advice on normal postural variations – intoeing (due to metatarsus adductus), bow-leggedness (genu varum) and lumbar lordosis (producing a protuberant abdomen).

Tiptoe walking can be normal, and is a feature of premature infants. It may additionally be an early sign of spastic diplegia, due to a tightening of Achilles' tendon.

Come to terms: types of abnormality

Malformation = structural defect of an organ or area
Deformation = abnormal form or position of a part due to compression
Disruption = breakdown of otherwise normal development process

Some simple rules when dealing with the painful, limping, orthopaedic or arthritic child are listed below.

Orthopaedic rules ... OK?
above all, don't hurt the child
active movements always before passive
never force a joint – especially a suspected congenital dislocation of hip
if in doubt, don't!

Come to terms: orthopaedic	
talipes equino varus = club foot	
genu varum	= bow-legged
genu valgum	= knock-kneed
genu recurvation	= knees bent backwards
gibbus	= sharply angled kyphosis

The newborn

At this age one's major interest is in detection of congenital abnormality. Are there 10 fingers and 10 toes? Any webs? Are the limbs symmetrical? Any positional deformities? Mild positional deformities of the feet, for example, varus (inturning) or valgus (out-turning), are common. Gentle manipulation will restore the foot to its correct position.

Fixed deformities such as club foot (talipes equino varus) are frequently associated with spina bifida, and will not correct on manipulation.

Developmental dysplasia of the hip (see Newborn examination, Chapter 4)

The correct technique of the hip examination is important to acquire – the 'Baby Hippy' may help in this respect. It is vital to remember that if developmental dysplasia of the hip (DDH) is not detected in the newborn period, it may not be evident until walking is attempted, at which stage *curative* correction is difficult. Hip examination is rewarding in the first week, less so at 6 weeks, and unrewarding at 6 months. After the newborn period the major sign of DDH is limited abduction of the hip.

Come to terms: finger/toe	
syndactyly	= fusion of digits
clinodactyly	= incurved digit
camptodactyly	= flexed digit
polydactyly	= extra digits
arachnodactyly	= long thin digits

Limb deformities

Limb reduction defects (of the type seen following thalidomide ingestion in pregnancy) are rare and will not be considered in detail. Proper measurement of limb length will be valuable in suspected asymmetry. Precise measurement of the lower limb is from the anterior iliac spine to the lower aspect of the medial malleolus. Hemihypertrophy has important associations with, for example, aniridia (absence of the iris) and nephroblastoma.

Come to terms: limb deformities	
amelia	= absence of limb
hemimelia	= absence of distal half of limb
phocomelia	= hand or foot attached directly to trunk
arthrogryposis	= curved joints
osteogenesis imperfecta	= brittle bone disease (fragilitas ossium)

Neural tube defects are sufficiently common, particularly in Celtic races, to warrant mention. The defects are usually obvious on inspection, and the associated disabilities and deformities will depend on the site and size of the lesion. The length and width of the lesion should be measured. The different types of neural tube defects are encephalocele, myelomeningocele, meningocele, and spina bifida occulta or dysraphism. In the minor and lower spinal types of spina bifida the clinical signs may be subtle – hairy tuft overlying the spine, 'lipomatous' lump or mild lower limb wasting or weakness. There is a strong association between neural tube defect and hydrocephalus.

Spina bifida occulta describes an incomplete fusion of vertebral arches on radiographs.

Come to terms: neural tube defects

spina bifida	= failure of fusion of vertebral arches (synonym = rachischisis)
meningocele	= open vertebral arches with overlying sac containing cerebrospinal fluid
myelomeningocele	= unfused vertebral arches with exposed neural tissue
hydranencephaly	= almost complete absence of cerebral hemispheres
anencephaly	= congenital absence of cranial vault
encephalocele	= herniation of brain through congenital skull defect

---

The neck

An apparent short neck is common in the newborn. Normal neck movement can be demonstrated by turning the baby's head to 90° on each side.

A fibrous nodule midway along the sternomastoid muscle (sternomastoid 'tumour') is an occasional finding in the neonate. It usually resolves spontaneously.

The thyroid gland is usually neither visible nor palpable in the newborn. An obvious goitre suggests some form of hypothyroidism (secondary to a thyroid enzyme deficiency) or transient hyperthyroidism.

Thyroglossal cysts are rare midline lesions which change position with tongue movement.

Toddler and preschool child

The normal toddler frequently has a mildly bow-legged gait. This may convert to a knock-kneed posture in the preschool age. Neither should cause concern unless extreme. Most toddlers have flat feet. Intoeing is a frequent finding due usually to metatarsus varus or to tibial torsion.

Limp

Limp is a frequent clinical problem in small children and will require careful examination of spine, hip, knee and foot.

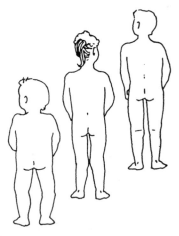

Fig. 5.30 Normal lower limb variations.

The approach to the limping child will be based on (a) history, (b) age and (c) clinical examination. The chronology of hip disorders in children has been well described. Inspection of the child's position, gait and lower limb will be imperative. Examination of hip, knee and ankle joint for range of movement will follow. A careful search for local heat or tenderness, for embedded foreign body, and for rash or lumps will be necessary. Among the multiple causes of acute limp in a child one could include the following:

- irritable hip
- transient synovitis
- pyogenic arthritis
- osteomyelitis
- discitis
- osteochondritis
- puncture wound, verruca, foreign body in foot
- spiral fracture of tibia or fibula

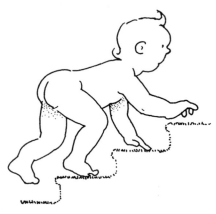

Fig. 5.31 Toddler climbing steps.

- rheumatoid arthritis
- bone tumour
- trauma
- Perthes' disease
- slipped femoral epiphysis
- anaphylactoid purpura
- lymphatic leukaemia
- coagulation disorder
- inguinal hernia
- testicular torsion.

Musculo-skeletal system

The term orthopaedics literally means 'straight child'. The term paediatrics means 'child doctor'. We once heard an illuminating lecture entitled 'Paediatrics as orthopaedic medicine', which cleverly combined the words and concepts. Children are brought to doctors to have their malformations corrected (if possible), their broken bones fixed (frequently) and their aches and pains relieved. Accidents and injuries are now the commonest reason for children's attendance at and admission to hospitals. As a result the orthopaedic department can be the busiest in the hospital. We are firm believers that, as implied in the lecture title above, orthopaedic surgeons and paediatric physicians should work closely together.

Needless to remark, the examination of muscles and nerves are inter-related exercises. Likewise, examination of muscles and joints must be integrated. The subdivisions between the chapters on nerves, muscles and joints are somewhat artificial and arbitrary, and they should best be seen as a continuum. No muscle or joint is an island unto itself and lesions are often multiple rather than isolated.

Muscles

Muscle disorder in childhood may reflect neurological diseases or intrinsic muscle disease, more likely the former. Early clues to neuromuscular disorder include reduced intrauterine activity, postnatal respiratory distress, floppiness, poor sucking and swallowing, and delayed developmental milestones. Later, an affected child may be slow to walk, poorly coordinated and clumsy, tire easily (wish to be carried everywhere), or fall often.

Examination of muscles includes inspection, palpation, testing muscle strength and excluding neurological disorder.

Muscle inspection. Here one is primarily concerned with size and symmetry. Absence or hypoplasia of a muscle group is recognized in certain syndromes – the angle of the mouth in congenital heart disease, the pectoralis major in Poland's syndrome, and the abdominal muscles in 'prune belly' syndrome.

Unilateral joint disease (say of the knee) may result in unilateral muscle wasting (of the quadriceps). It is well worth noting the degree of muscle wasting which can follow prolonged immobilization of a child's limb in a fracture cast.

Hypertrophy of muscle groups may imply physical use (swimmers have strong shoulder muscles). Some children with certain short-limbed bone disorders look strikingly muscular. The legs of children with hypochondroplasia or achondroplasia may appear to be 'muscular'. The calf muscles may appear large, but feel rubbery, in Duchenne's muscular dystrophy.

Palpation of muscles. Muscle tenderness is indicative of myositis. Acute viral myositis with refusal to walk, tenderness of the calf muscles, and little constitutional upset is a recognized clinical entity. It is seen usually in children aged 5–10 years. Influenza virus and Coxsackie virus infections may cause myalgia (muscle pain) in children but not usually myositis. Muscle pain and tenderness are well recognized features of ascending polyneuritis (Guillain–Barré syndrome) in children. Muscle tenderness is seen in dermatomyositis, a rare childhood condition. We have only once felt the vermiform mass of visceral larva migrans but suspect it may be more common in developing countries. Muscle tumours (such as myosarcoma) or bone tumours (such as osteosarcoma or chondrosarcoma) are rare in childhood, but may present as masses, apparently in or adherent to muscle groups.

Muscle strength. This can be difficult to determine in preschool children, but should be easily assessable in schoolchildren. Students are not expected to know the relative strength of various groups of muscles at different ages. One arbitrary method of grading strength is shown in Table 5.12.

If the truth be told most of us ordinary mortals and paediatricians require the assistance of a physiotherapist or neurologist to accurately grade and gauge the strength of groups of muscles.

A couple of simple screening tests may be helpful and illustrative. Think of yourself – what movements would you do if asked to test the strength of your calf muscles (stand on your toes?), biceps (lift a litre of beer?), or abdominal

Table 5.12 An arbitrary method for grading strength		
Grade	Crude assessment	Degree of weakness
0	None	No movement
1	Minimal	Flicker of movement
2	Poor	Movement with gravity only
3	Fair	Movement against gravity
4	Good	Mild weakness
5	Normal	Normal

muscles (do a sit-up?). Now apply your common sense to small children.

- Lift toddler up under his arms – tests proximal muscles of upper limbs.
- Hold toddler by fingertips – tests distal arm muscles.
- Ask toddler to crawl up steps – tests proximal and distal muscles of lower limbs.
- Ask toddler/child to get up from sitting position. This tests the calf muscles. Gower's sign (where the child 'climbs up' his legs) is a classic sign of muscular dystrophy but is seen in other forms of muscle weakness.
- Ask the child to squeeze your two fingers – 'hurt me if you can'. They usually enjoy this. Tests grip strength.
- Ask the child to pull your hair (with fingers only) – they really enjoy this! Tests small hand muscles.

We could go on but trust you have got the message. Play games, indulge in mock fights, pit your strength against theirs, be encouraging and positive:

'Let's see how strong you are.'
'Come on! You can do better than that.'

Most boys enjoy these exercises and modern girls are not far behind.

Schoolchild

In this section we propose to mention selectively (a) joint examination, (b) arthritis and (c) examination for scoliosis.

The systematic examination of muscles, joints and bones in the schoolchild is as for an adult. Limb or joint pain is a common symptom seeking explanation. The term 'arthralgia' means joint pain. It is important to ascertain from the parents of a child with limb pain its periodicity, precipitating and relieving events and, most importantly, whether or not they have noticed any swelling or redness in the affected part.

All students must be able to examine all joints, but particularly (a) the hand, (b) the hip and (c) the knee, these being the joints most commonly involved in arthritic process.

Joint examination

Arthritis, or joint inflammation, is a common phenomenon in paediatrics. It may occur in rubella (affecting the knees especially), in infectious mononucleosis, in Henoch–Schönlein syndrome (affecting the large joints), fleetingly in rheumatic fever (which 'licks the joints and bites the heart'), in collagen-vascular disorders such as systemic lupus erythematosus, and in the various chronic arthritides of childhood. Arthritis is manifest by the presence of the classic signs of inflammation:

- rubor (redness)
- calor (heat)
- dolor (pain)
- tumour (swelling)
- functiolasia (loss of function).

Joints may also be involved in infectious processes. Septic arthritis may involve hips or knees. Tuberculous arthritis commonly used to involve hips and spines, but is no longer common in the Western world. Meningococcaemia may be accompanied by joint infection.

Joints may be damaged or their function disordered by congenital malformation, as in arthrogryposis multiplex, or acetabular dysplasia, now thought to be a common association with dislocated hips.

Pain is the primary complaint in arthritis. Children are brought to doctors for (a) relief of pain, (b) suppression of inflammation or infection, (c) maintenance of joint position

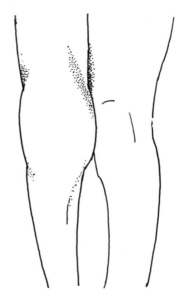

Fig. 5.32 Swollen arthritic knee.

and function and (d) prevention of deformity. The primary objective in joint examination is to achieve an anatomical, pathological and functional diagnosis leading to appropriate management. In simple terms, one wants to know what joints are affected, how badly and for what reason.

Finally, arthralgia and arthritis may be due to trauma, bleeding disorder (factor 8 or 9 deficiency), or to one of the many eponymic osteochondritides, such as Osgood–Schlatter disease. In small pre-vocal infants and toddlers, joint pain may be manifest by unwillingness to move a limb, or by crying when being bathed or changed. A mother recently said of her infant with Still's disease: 'I just could not touch him but he cried'.

Correct examination of any joint depends on:

- inspection and accurate description of observations
- palpation for heat, tenderness, swelling and crepitus
- testing range of movement.

The basic rules of examination are look first, palpate gently without hurting and always do active movements before passive movements. The gait should be routinely observed. 'Growing pains' are a misnomer – physical growth is not painful, but 'psychological growth can hurt like hell'.

Joint inspection involves looking for the presence of joint swelling, for loss of usual bony landmarks and joint contours, and for associated muscle wasting. Joint swelling may be due to synovial thickening or joint effusion or both. In the knee, wrist and interphalangeal joints, swelling may be obvious. The purpuric rash of Henoch–Schönlein syndrome may accompany obvious arthritis of the ankle and knee, making diagnosis simple. Swollen interphalangeal joints produce a spindle-shaped deformity of the fingers. Swelling of the wrist joint may result in a 'dinner-fork' deformity. Swelling of shoulder and hip joints is not usually visible.

Joint palpation implies a search for joint heat using the palm or back of one's hand according to preference. One must compare joint heat with its pair and with surrounding structures. Obvious joint heat strongly suggests an inflammatory arthritis. Joint tenderness may be assessed by gently pressing, compressing or squeezing the joint. Joint swelling due to synovial thickening can be best appreciated at the wrist where the thickened synovium may be palpable. Joint effusion is easiest to detect at the knee joint. With a small amount of fluid in the knee the bulge sign can mobilize the fluid between various pouches. A large amount of fluid in the knee joint is indicated by a positive patellar tap.

Joint movement. Testing joint movement requires a knowledge of the normal range of movement of a given major joint – about 180° at the wrist and 140° at the knee, for example. It is beyond the remit of this text to list ranges of movement of flexion, extension, rotation or abduction of various joints at different ages. An infant can get his toe into his mouth; most adults can only achieve this with training or torture. You should know the normal ranges at ankle, knee, hip, wrist, elbows, shoulders and neck joints (see Table 5.13).

Finally, a word of caution. Always perform active movements before passive movements. Doing things the other way round may result in you hurting the child. If you hurt a child during examination, and he cries – end of examination, upset child, angry mother, failed student?

The term 'juvenile idiopathic arthritis' (JIA) is now used to describe the various chronic arthritides of childhood. Sir Frederick Still elegantly described a cluster of conditions, emphasizing the systemic nature of the condition in the young child involving skin, glands, spleen, liver and bone marrow, as well as the joints.

Table 5.13 Normal range of movement at various joints		
Joint	Movement	Normal range
Wrist	Flexion	90°
	Extension	90°
Elbow	Flexion	0–15°
	Extension	0–15°
Knees	Flexion	30°
	Hyperextension	0–5°
Ankle	Dorsiflexion	30°
	Plantar flexion	30°

Classification of juvenile idiopathic arthritis

Definition of JIA: arthritis present for 6 or more weeks for which no other cause can be found.

Subtypes

1. Oligoarticular onset JIA: fewer than five joints involved during the first 6 months of disease.
   Persistent: four or fewer total joints involved during the duration of follow-up.
   Extended: more than four joints involved during duration of follow-up.
2. Polyarticular onset JIA: five or more joints involved during first 6 months of disease, usually involving small joints in a symmetrical distribution.

Rheumatoid factor negative/positive.

3. Systemic onset JIA (formerly known as Still's disease): chronic arthritis associated with systemic features including high spiking fevers, transient episodic erythematous rash, lymphadenopathy and hepatosplenomegaly.
4. Psoriatic arthritis: chronic arthritis usually with asymmetric small and large joint involvement, and either the development of psoriasis or other evidence of a psoriatic diathesis (family history, nail pits).
5. Enthesitis-related arthritis: previously known as juvenile spondyloarthropathy. Chronic arthritis associated with enthesitis (inflammation at insertion of tendons, ligaments or fascia to bone), or with lower axial skeletal involvement. An HLA-B27-related arthropathy. A significant proportion of patients will develop sacroiliitis as adults, but back and sacroiliac joint involvement is uncommon during childhood.
6. Unclassified: any form of idiopathic chronic arthritis that does not fit into the above categories.

Come to terms: painful words

myalgia	= muscle pain
arthralgia	= joint pain
neuralgia	= nerve pain
proctalgia	= rectal pain
migraine	= unilateral headache (hemi-crania = half head)

Scoliosis

Routine examination, particularly in adolescent schoolgirls, should include inspection for scoliosis. Scoliosis is sought by:

1. Inspection from behind in the upright posture. One shoulder may be elevated and the lumbar or thoracic spine may apparently be curved. It is usual to describe the curvature on the basis of its convexity (to right or left).
2. Asking the child to touch her toes. The examiner should be seated behind the child with eyes horizontal to the bent back. A fixed scoliosis will be evidenced by a hump. A postural scoliosis will correct on bending.

Hip ages

birth:	CHD/DDH
1–3 years:	transient synovitis
5 years:	Perthes' disease
10 years:	slipped epiphysis
any age:	inflammatory arthritis

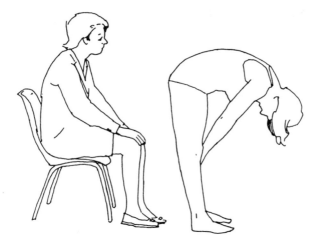

Fig. 5.33 Inspecting for scoliosis.

THE EYES

The eye is the window of the soul.

The eyes can tell a lot about all of us. When indulging in the art of physiognomy (attempting to assess character from facial features) one first looks at the eyes. So too in children. The dull, sunken eyes in dehydration; the sad, depressed eyes in marasmic malnutrition; the yellow sclera of jaundice; the pink iris of albinism; the bright, sparkling eyes of gaiety and good health.

Eye examination should include:

- general inspection of the eye, pupil, iris, sclera
- assessment of eye movement, with a comment on symmetry or otherwise
- pupillary, accommodation and corneal reflexes as appropriate
- red reflex

- retinal funduscopy (with the ophthalmoscope)
- assessment of visual acuity.

Ophthalmoscopy

Good ophthalmoscopy is an integral part of examination of any child, irrespective of age. In the newborn, assistance is required to hold the head correctly in the midline. The eyelids can be gently prised apart. Elicit the red reflex in both eyes from a distance of 20 cm. Inspect the cornea for clarity, seek any lens opacity and examine the fundus to detect haemorrhages, retinopathy and appearance of the disc.

Funduscopy can be very difficult in toddlers and pre-school children. Keep the infant or child in his position of comfort – lying, sitting on his mother's knee or sitting alone. Darken the room if necessary. Keep the light intensity of the ophthalmoscope down. Do not use mydriatics (without permission). Try to get the child to look at an attractive but distracting object. Do not force the eyes open – this usually results in resistance and rejection. Be patient, approaching slowly from a distance. Patience and perseverance may be rewarded by the recognition of an identifiable retinopathy (for example rubella, cytomegalovirus or toxoplasma retinopathy in a child whose handicaps were previously unexplained).

Other rare findings include: retinopathy of prematurity (retrolental fibroplasia), hypertensive retinopathy, choroidal tubercle, *Toxocara* (ocular larva migrans). Papilloedema is rare in the presence of open fontanellae and sutures.

Funduscopy findings

- rubella retinopathy = 'pepper and salt' appearance on retina (rare)

- toxoplasmosis   = one or many pigmented or atrophic scars (rare)
- cherry-red spot   = seen in a variety of rare inherited disorders (rare).

In infants and children always first ask the mother: 'Does your child see well?' If she replies 'yes', ask her to tell you her reasons. She's usually right. If she thinks her child sees poorly, seek the reason. The onus lies on the doctor to determine whether she's right or wrong.

Occasional eye findings of no consequence

1. *Pseudostrabismus* (pseudosquint) is the spurious appearance of a squint due to broad nasal bridge or prominent epicanthic folds.
2. *Blue sclerae* are usually normal in infancy. Strikingly blue sclerae are seen in osteogenesis imperfecta, in inherited connective tissue disorders and occasionally in iron deficiency.
3. *Blinking* is often a form of habit spasm or tic in schoolchildren, and is best ignored.
4. *Light reflection* is useful at all ages. Light from a distant source (the window, a light bulb, or torch) should fall symmetrically on the pupils or iris through all ranges of movements.

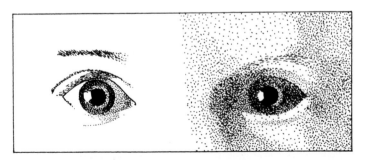

Fig. 5.34 Light reflection is useful at all ages.

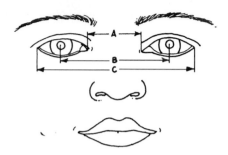

Fig. 5.35 Ocular landmarks: A = inner-canthal distance, B = interpupillary distance, C = outer canthal distance.

Normal values for ocular landmarks (Fig. 5.35) can be found in specialized texts. Hypertelorism exists when the eyes are widely spaced apart.

The term 'mongoloid slant' is used when the eyes slope upwards and outwards. By converse, 'anti-mongoloid slant' is downwards and outwards.

Observational ophthalmology

We have stressed throughout this text the rewards of careful observation. A good look at the eyes is well worthwhile.

1. *Cataract* may be seen. Cataracts are associated with congenital rubella and galactosaemia.
2. *Corneal clouding* may be apparent. This is suggestive of mucopolysaccharidosis.
3. *Nystagmus* may be noted.
4. Roving, purposeless eye movements with little visual fixation are typical of the infant with visual impairment.
5. *Ptosis* of the eyelid may be obvious.
6. Males with the fragile X syndrome have cold (often blue) piercing eyes.

7. The 'frozen watchfulness' of the battered or abused child may be observed. His gaze is calculated and seems to go through you.
8. *Leukocoria* = absence of red reflex. This may indicate retinoblastoma, cataract or retinopathy of prematurity.

Come to terms: eyes

amblyopia	= 'lazy' eye; partial loss of vision
aniridia	= congenital absence of the iris
anophthalmia	= congenital absence of the eye (orbit)
aphakia	= congenital absence of the lens

A few simple points to remember about eye examination are that:

- children do not like having their eyes prised open
- accommodation is strong in preschool children
- pupillary inequality is an occasional normal finding

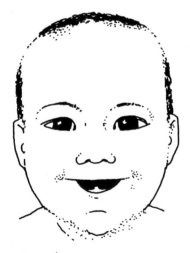

Fig. 5.36 A responsive smile.

- symmetry of movement, colour and reaction is important to establish.

Eye examination at different ages

Newborn

Neonates dislike strong light; however, turning to light is a useful clinical test during the first month. Transitory fixation may be elicited by bringing a red (ball) object into the visual field at a distance of about 30–50 cm.

The newborn's eyes are best examined with the baby upright, and, if necessary, sucking. They will usually open in this position. With patience and a cooperative baby you may see the baby's eyes 'lock' onto his mother's.

At birth, examination is mainly to exclude gross abnormalities, evidence of possible trauma and congenital or acquired infection. Eye movement at this stage is established through the use of the vestibular ocular reflex, where rotating the baby from side to side, backwards and forwards and up and down will elicit eye movements in all directions.

Disconjugate movements may be present in the first week or two but are usually gone by 4 weeks. Eye size should be checked to exclude eyes that are too big (glaucoma) or too small (microphthalmia). The cornea should be perfectly clear within 1 or 2 days after birth. The pupils should be equal and reactive. Always be suspicious of different coloured eyes at this stage.

Assessment of alignment is best carried out with an ophthalmoscope at about a distance of 0.5 m. At this distance the examiner can observe both pupils simultaneously and compare redness and brightness of the red reflex. If inequality of the redness occurs, the possibility of a strabismus or an opacity in the eye should be considered. Funduscopy at this stage shows occasional haemorrhages, particularly around the disc and posterior pole. If the haemorrhages are extensive, an ophthalmological opinion should be sought. Sometimes in the first few days, oedema of the eyelids causes difficulty in opening the eye for proper examination and in this case placing the baby in the prone position will facilitate eye opening.

6–8 weeks

The infant is alert to moving objects although convergence and following are jerky. An examiner can readily hold the infant's attention at a distance of about 30 cm and a rewarding smile 'with meaning' is elicited. By 12 weeks head and eye movements may be demonstrated through 180°. At this age lacrimal glands will show response to emotion.

16–20 weeks

Hand regard develops and a 2.5-cm (1-inch) brick will cause immediate fixation within a distance of 1 m. Colour preference develops from 20–28 weeks and hand/eye coordination (palmar grasp) can readily be elicited using brick or paper. Visual acuity continues to improve dramatically from 9 to 12 months and very small objects can be seen and picked up using index finger and thumb. There is smooth visual movement in both the horizontal and vertical planes. At 1 year the transverse diameter of the cornea is adult size (12 mm). Convergence is well established by 18 months. By the age of 4 years visual acuity is nearly 20/20.

Examination of the eyes should be carried out in every patient irrespective of age. Skill in the proper use of the ophthalmoscope should be acquired early in clinical training. Assessment should occur in the neonatal period, at the toddler stage (2–3 years) and again at 5 years (preschool). Subsequently to this, assessment should be carried out every 2–3 years to late teens.

Strabismus (squint)

Parents will often offer the opinion that their child has a squint. Squint may be more apparent when the child is tired. Relatives or friends may point out a squint to the parents. Students should always accept parents' opinion concerning squint and test the eyes appropriately. Squint in the newborn is not significant so long as you can exclude a retinoblastoma. Approach squints in the following fashion:

1. Look for light reflection through all movements.
2. Test eye movement and muscles in all directions. A simple method of checking all eye movements is to draw an imaginary 'Union Jack' in the air while asking the child to follow your finger (Fig. 5.37).
3. Try to answer the simple question – is this squint alternating (concomitant) or paralytic?
4. Look for corneal opacities and cataracts.
5. Do the cover test. Use an interesting object (toy) to hold the child's attention. The eye is covered on the visual axis to make viewing of the object monocular. If the child has been fixing with the eye just covered, the other eye will take over fixation in the presence of a squint.

Any squint persisting beyond 5–6 months from birth is significant and should be referred immediately to an ophthalmologist. Pseudosquint is a common minor variation. Paralytic squint, though rare, tends to have more serious connotations than alternating squint.

Come to terms: eye lumps	
chalazion	= small inclusion cyst in eyelid
hordeolum	= stye in the eyelid (pustule)
dermoid	= external angle dermoid of eye
pinguecula	= small yellowish patch near the cornea

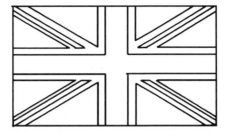

Fig. 5.37 The Union Jack.

The red reflex

Shine a light at both eyes from a distance of 0.5 m. There should be a symmetrical red reflex. A white pupillary reflex will be caused by cataract, retinoblastoma and retinopathy of prematurity. Absence of the red reflex is called leukocoria.

Occasional eye findings

1. *Dilated conjunctival vessels* may suggest ataxia – telangiectasia.
2. *Brushfield's spots* (white spots around the outer iris) are seen in Down's syndrome but also in normal children.
3. *Morgan–Dennie fold* is a double fold under the eye. It is seen in eczematous, allergic children.

The neurological examination and interpretation of the eyes are similar in children and adults. Pupils should normally be equal, central, circular and respond to light and accommodation. Eye movements should be full in all directions. Fine nystagmus on extreme deviation is a normal finding. The corneal reflex is unpleasant and rarely needs to be elicited. We will not detail testing of visual acuity at different ages – refer to Mary Sheridan's book (1997) or to a textbook of ophthalmology. In cooperative children, visual fields can be roughly assessed by confrontation tests.

In early infancy the following may be warning signs of poor visual activity
roving or wandering eye movements
persistence of hand regard
lack of blink to a hand thrust rapidly toward the face ('blinking to menace')
nystagmus

Early detection and treatment of squint can prevent amblyopia. Early detection of reduced visual acuity can lead to appropriate therapy.

At all clinic visits ask the mother:

Can your baby see well?
Tell me why you think so.

If she's worried about her baby's vision, take her on her word. Her insight is usually right! Remember that infants fix readily on mothers' eyes and like best to look at friendly smiling human faces in preference to pens, stethoscopes, or other dangling objects. A familiar doll or toy may complement your smile!

SURGERY

This section describes observation and examination for conditions requiring either immediate or later surgery.

1. **Inguinal hernia** – is most commonly found in the first 3 months, more particularly in preterm infants. In the vast majority of cases a male infant is affected, though very rarely a female infant can present with the same condition. A preterm infant should not be allowed home before surgery, as strangulation is a very real possibility. Association with examination for hernia should include the presence and position of testes. Cold hands and a crying infant can make

this assessment difficult and result in an uncertain diagnosis. Warm hands and a soother (teat) can be very helpful.

2. **Umbilical hernia** – common in infancy and more common in the preterm. Umbilical hernias are easily reducible. By putting your little finger in the hernia, you may feel the small defect in the linea alba. Most umbilical hernias resolve spontaneously. Umbilical hernia is very unlikely ever to become an emergency.

3. **Torsion of testis** (one or both). This condition is rare and usually occurs prior to birth. Examination in the first 48 hours will reveal a large hard discoloured testis, which over the following weeks will disintegrate and disappear. If the condition is unilateral, early stabilization of the remaining testis is urgent.

4. **Ear examination.** Rarely an acute middle ear infection with bulging drum may require the early intervention of an otological surgeon and rarer still an acute mastoiditis. Where there is evidence of middle ear infection on examination – always palpate the mastoid process for tenderness.

5. **Tonsils.** Very occasionally tonsils may become so acutely enlarged that they require otological intervention. However, the most infected-looking tonsils with a pustular covering are more likely to be a result of glandular fever – a benign condition.

6. **Ingrown toe nail.** A great majority of neonates and infants have what appears to be ingrown toe nails. Staphylococcal infections can produce paronychia. Surgery is rarely, if ever, indicated as local therapy resolves.

7. **Acute osteomyelitis.** This is not an uncommon condition and, where being considered, a careful examination for a localized area of acute pain and tenderness is necessary. Happily, surgery is very rarely necessary now.

8. **Acute appendicitis.** This is a notoriously difficult condition to diagnose in young children. Though one has seen an occasional case in infancy, it is far more common in older

schoolchildren. The abdomen should be carefully examined for localized pain. Be very gentle. Warm hands are essential. If possible a parent should be present to relax and console the child. If in doubt, help from a more senior colleague is essential. Where possible perforation is being considered, a rectal examination and abdominal scan may be helpful in confirming the diagnosis.

9. **Periorbital infection.** This is where you observe inflammation and oedema in the periorbital skin and underlying tissues. This is an emergency condition and immediate ophthalmological opinion is recommended.

10. **Pyloric stenosis.** The signs are visible peristalsis over the stomach and a palpable pyloric tumour or mass. The pyloric tumour is in the right upper quadrant and feels like an olive (or the tip of your nose). It is best felt as a part of a 'test feed' but is not easy to palpate.

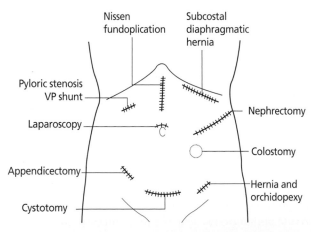

Fig. 5.38 Some abdominal scars seen in children. Please note that many of these operations are now performed laparoscopically.

6 A measure of progress

A paediatrician is a measuring doctor.

Apley

Chesterton has stated that the man who knew him best was his tailor, for he measured him afresh each time he met him. The same should be said of children's doctors, who should habitually measure length (height), weight and head circumference of all infants and toddlers. In addition, arm circumference, skinfold thickness, blood pressure, upper-lower segment ratios, etc., will be measured as appropriate.

In infancy, lying length is measured. Most crudely this can be done by measuring crown–heel length using a tape. More accurate methods are horizontal stadiometers or the 'pedobaby' measurer. Standing height can be measured against simple wall charts, against vertical rulers, or using a stadiometer (Fig. 6.1). The most accurate methods have been established by Tanner's group. Height should ideally

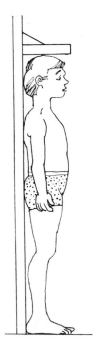

Fig. 6.1 Measuring height with stadiometer.

be plotted on a centile chart appropriate for sex, age and race. In early age (up to 7 years) there is little sex difference. International charts have been published. Height increment is probably a better indicator of well-being than weight gain.

In assessing children's height a number of simple ages are useful (see box).

Simple ages for assessing height

chronological (actual) age. Example: boy, age 6.0 years, measuring 100 cm

height age = 4 years. In other words, the boy is the same height as an average 4-year-old

bone age as assessed radiologically. This boy's bone age is assessed as 4 years with usual variation

clothes age. Mother reports buying clothes marked for a 4-year-old

---

Useful adjuncts in assessing growth and development:

- Ask to see child health record if parents have one
- Inspect family photographs regarding relative weight and height
- Enquire about familial traits –
  Was his father late into puberty?
  When did her mother's periods begin?

Height reference points

birth:	50 cm
1 year:	75 cm
4 years:	100 cm
12–13 years:	150 cm

It has been said in the Bible that a just *weight* is the Lord's delight and a false balance an abomination; so too in paediatrics. All babies, infants and toddlers need to be weighed regularly. Drug dosages and fluid requirements are related to body weight. In the first year of life, weight will increase threefold, length by 50% and head circumference by approximately one-third.

Head circumference, or more correctly, maximal occipito-frontal diameter, should also be measured using a nonstretchable and reliable tape (Fig. 6.2). Head circumference is an indicator of brain growth (but not of intelligence). One is looking for heads which are growing unusually rapidly or unusually slowly. In ordinary practice one usually defines the upper and lower third centiles (which are equivalent to ± 2 SD) as the borders of 'normality' (Fig. 6.3). Measurements less than the third centile do not necessarily imply abnormality: many of these will be 'small normals'.

Average head circumference	
birth:	35 cm
1 year:	47 cm
2 years:	49 cm
4 years:	50 cm
8 years:	52 cm
15 years:	55 cm

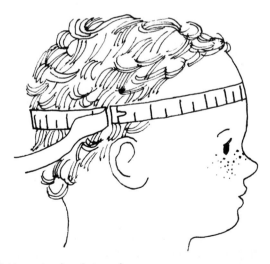

Fig. 6.2 Measuring head circumference.

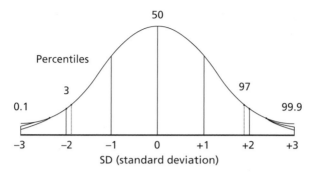

Fig. 6.3 Relation between centiles and standard deviations.

Height and head circumference, for example, do run in families. Cognizance of parents' height must always be taken in assessment of short stature. Charts for equating children's height with mid-parental height are available. Familial macrocephaly is a well-recognized entity – parental head circumference measurement is an essential part of the assessment of any infant or child with an unusually large head.

Other useful measurements include:

1. *Arm span*: from fingertip to fingertip, across shoulders. This should approximate standing height from age 3–4 years. If less than height it may suggest short limbs.
2. *Upper-lower segment ratio*: the measurements are from pubis to crown, and from pubis to ground. In the schoolchild the ratio is close to unity. It is 1.7:1 in the newborn.
3. *Arm circumference*: halfway between the shoulder and the elbow. In developing countries this is a useful index of nutrition.
4. *Skinfold thickness*: using an appropriate caliper. Measurements are usually made in the left mid-triceps region and in the left subscapular area and are used to gauge under- and overnutrition.

5. Height (and weight) *velocity*, which measures the rate of change as opposed to the distance achieved.
6. *Body mass index* (BMI): weight (kg) ÷ height (m²). Normal is 18–25. BMI is a useful index of obesity in childhood.

Catch-up growth: 8-year-old boy

chronological age = 8 years
height age   = 4 years
bone age   = 4 years
clothes age   = 4–5 years

  coeliac disease diagnosed at age 8 years
  catch-up growth demonstrated thereafter on gluten-free diet.

Somebody has measured just about everything imaginable relating to children – interpupillary distance, stretched penile length, testicular volume, kidney size, cardiothoracic ratio – and their normal values can be obtained from specialized texts. With regard to height:

• plot on centile charts
• serial measurements are more important than single ones
• patterns of aberrant growth are well recognized
• children tend to stick to centile channels.

In approaching the unusually small or tall child, simple questions, accurate measurements and appropriate centile and velocity chartings will often save a lot of time and much unnecessary investigation. A typical algorithm for approaching the small child is shown in Fig. 6.4.

If there are no previous measurements on a small child, his mother should be asked about shoe size, clothes size and age (many large stores label clothes by age), and you could ask to inspect family photographs. Although doctors

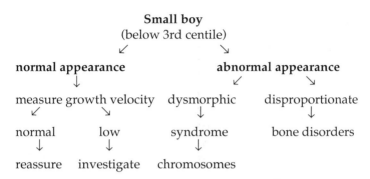

Fig. 6.4 Algorithm for approaching a boy in the third centile.

may be concerned about a small child, his mother may be nonplussed since 'all my family were slow starters'.

Children, especially boys, are conscious of their height and earnestly wish to match their peers. We don't entirely agree with the 'bottom line' in the following little poem:

I met a little Elfman once,
Down where the lilies blow,
I asked him why he was so small,
And why he did not grow.
He slightly frowned and with his eyes,
He looked me through and through.
'I'm quite as big enough for me', he said,
'As you are big for you'.

John K Bangs

Finally, some simple pointers:

- centile charts describe what is, not what should be
- there may be a significant difference in height between the best and worse off segments in society, but not necessarily in weight

- most small children are 'small normal' children coming from families of small parents and/or from socially deprived groups
- there is probably nothing wrong with those small children (below third centile) who demonstrate normal growth velocity observed over 6–12 months
- static height or weight in a child is unusual and may be a sign of disease
- crossing down centile channels is abnormal.

Come to terms: short stature	
diastrophic dwarfism	= crooked dwarfism
thanatophoric dwarfism	= death-bearing dwarfism
achondroplasia	= a form of short-limbed dwarfism
osteopetrosis	= marble bone disease

We believe that students need not spend too much time on rare and unusual cases, however interesting they may be. If you can stimulate the skill of recognizing what's different, if you can describe what you see, and if you know suitable sources of further information, that should suffice.

Dysmorphology depends on recognition, description and measurement. One can consult appropriate texts or a suitably programmed computer.

The *measurements used in dysmorphology* include:

- height
- arm span
- upper-lower segment ratios
- hand length
- metacarpal length
- ear length
- interocular distance
- forearm carrying angle
- inner canthal distance
- bone age.

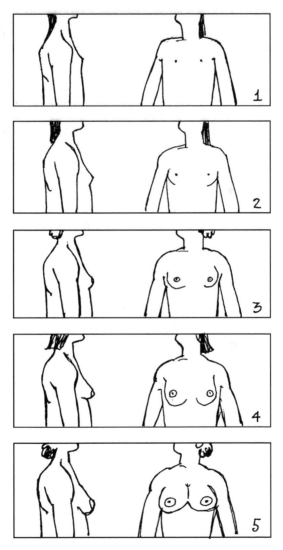

Fig. 6.5 The five stages of female breast development.

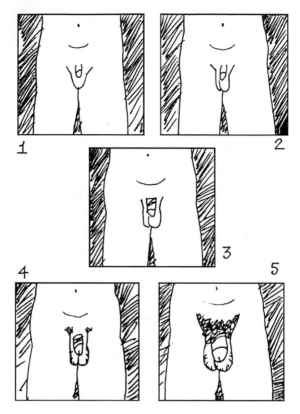

Fig. 6.6 The five stages of male genital and pubic hair development.

In prepubertal and pubertal children, assessment of puberty status can be helpful. Directions for assessing puberty status are given in Tanner–Whitehouse (UK growth standards) and are based on breast, genital and pubic hair growth.

7 Hydration and nutrition

DETECTING AND DETERMINING DEHYDRATION

In maintaining normal hydration, infants are dependent on their attendants (mother, nurse, etc.) to supply a sufficient quantity of fluid. For a variety of physiological and practical reasons, dehydration can arise easily and rapidly in infancy. Early detection and determination of the degree of dehydration is therefore essential.

Why is dehydration common in infants?

1. Infants have a different body composition to adults – 70–80% body water content versus 60% in adults.
2. High fluid intake – 150 ml/kg/day compared with 30–40 ml/kg/day in adults.
3. Daily water turnover of 10–15% of body weight compared with 3–5% in adults.

4. Relative reduction in renal ability to concentrate urine.
5. Greater surface area/mass ratio, resulting in high insensible fluid losses through skin and respiratory tract. Factor X2–3.
6. Higher basal metabolic rate plus greater febrile response to infection.
7. Infants have little or no control over fluid intake.

A normal state of hydration is manifest by bright eyes, moist tongue and good skin turgor. Fat infants (in whom skin turgor is difficult to determine) may deceive by concealing dehydration, especially of the hypertonic type. Appreciation of normal skin turgor or elasticity is best established by examining lots of normal infants.

Signs of dehydration

Dehydration in infancy is manifested by:

1. A sunken anterior fontanelle
2. Dull, dry eyes with reduced eyeball turgor (as most of us do not normally assess eyeball turgor in normal infants, one can be uncertain of this sign)
3. Dry tongue and mouth
4. Diminished skin turgor or elasticity, which is best elicited by picking up abdominal or thigh skin (Fig. 7.1)
5. Lethargy and weak cry
6. Diminished pulse volume
7. Diminished urinary output (more dry nappies)
8. Reduced blood pressure.

It is important to remember that the early signs of dehydration reflect loss of interstitial fluid volume, whereas the later signs (Nos. 6–8) reflect loss of intravascular volume. Most infants in developed countries get to medical attention when their dehydration is of a mild to moderate degree. In developing countries severe dehydration is a frequent

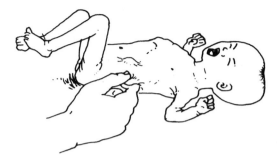

Fig. 7.1 Loss of normal skin turgor.

phenomenon. Infants with dehydration of the common isotonic or hypotonic variety are usually lethargic and 'flat'. By contrast hypertonic or hypernatraemic dehydration, which introduces a cerebral component to the illness, may be suspected if the infant is irritable or cranky.

Very severe dehydration may be accompanied by a metabolic acidosis (deep sighing respiration) or by shock (pallid, cold, quiet infant).

The figures in Table 7.1 highlight the important differences in fluid balance between the neonate, infant and adult. It must be emphasized that these are 'typical' values and that there is much variation.

Types of dehydration	
isotonic:	70%; flat, lethargic
hypotonic:	20–30%
hypertonic:	2–5%; irritable, 'doughy' skin, convulsion

It can be difficult to clinically determine the type of dehydration. It is important to be alert and to try to detect hypertonic dehydration, as this may result in convulsion and brain damage.

Table 7.1 Fluid facts

	1 week	1 year	20 years
Weight (kg)	3.0	10.0	70.0
Length (cm)	50	75	175
Head circumference (cm)	35	47	55
Body surface area (m²)	0.25	0.5	1.73
Blood pressure (mmHg)	70/40	90/50	120/80
Fluid intake (l/day)	0.45	1.0	2.5
Fluid intake (% body weight)	15	10	3.5
Fluid intake (ml/kg/day)	150	100	35
Blood volume (ml)	250	750	5000

The degree of dehydration

mild (< 5% loss of body weight) = few clinical signs. Perhaps dry tongue, flattish fontanelle

moderate (5–10% loss of body weight) = obvious clinical signs of loss of interstitial fluid – sunken fontanelle, dry tongue, reduced skin turgor

severe (10–15% loss of body weight) = seriously ill. Signs of loss of intravascular volume – weak, fast pulse, low blood pressure, poor urine output – plus earlier signs

Could we propose that the concept of body spaces is useful in understanding body fluids. There are three body fluid spaces: the first, second and third. We have always thought that it is very difficult to define the 'third world' when you are uncertain where the 'first' and 'second' worlds are.

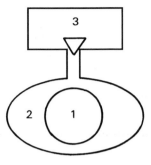

Fig. 7.2 The three fluid spaces.

first space   = the intravascular space
second space = interstitial space
third space   = fluid in pleural cavity, peritoneal cavity, gastrointestinal
                         tract, etc.

Fluid losses in the third space are concealed and may be unconsidered.

mild-moderate dehydration = ↓interstitial volume
severe dehydration   = ↓intravascular volume

Overhydration is less frequently encountered in children but may occur with cardiac failure, renal failure or excessive intravenous fluids. One might clinically attempt to estimate the degree of fluid overload (weight increase as a proportion of dry weight, if known) and aim to restore water balance by fluid restriction, diuretics or dialysis as appropriate. The cardinal clinical sign is oedema.

NUTRITION

Clinical assessment of nutrition is relatively simple. Modern Western infant malnutrition consists of children being fed the wrong foods (too much carbohydrate) and too many calories, resulting in obesity. In the developing world, protein, calorie, vitamin and mineral deficiencies are common. Inadequate food intake is a common cause of failure to thrive in all parts of the world.

Assessment of nutrition

- Look
- Weigh, measure and plot on centile chart
- Examination for specific deficiencies.

Observation

The well infant has full cheeks, firm rounded buttocks, good muscle tone and a healthy complexion. The infant's buttocks are like the camel's hump – a storage space of fat and muscle for hard times. Acute malnutrition in infancy manifests as weight loss, loose subcutaneous skin folds and apathy. Chronic malnutrition is evidenced by pallor, thinness, prominent bones, protuberant abdomen, hypotonia, flat buttocks and misery. The skin may be thin and shiny, the hair dull and lacklustre, and the nails brittle.

Weighing and measuring

This has been described in Chapter 6. Remember that centile charts describe what is, not what should be. They are gathered from normal children in a given population. Many of the children in the upper 'normal' centile ranges in Western populations look fat – they are fat.

Watch carefully those children who are crossing down centile lines.

The 'normal' thin child tends to have similar parents, to be active and sturdy, and to have proportionate height and weight centiles.

Growth is probably a better indicator of well-being than weight. Significant differences in height exist between the upper and lower social groups in most populations; weight differences may not be so evident.

Examination for specific deficiencies

Iron deficiency is the commonest type.

Anaemia. Inspect conjunctival mucous membrane, buccal mucous membrane, palmar creases, ear lobes and nailbeds for redness, or pallor. Use your own palms as controls (assuming you are not anaemic). Iron-deficient children are frequently unhappy or miserable. In Caucasian children facial pallor is more often a matter of skin complexion and lack of sunlight than of anaemia. However, healthy babies do have a good pink complexion. The clinical evaluation of anaemia is unreliable but worth attempting. Clinical signs of anaemia are usually not appreciable until the haemoglobin level is less than 10 g/dl (100 g/l). Obvious clinical signs should be expected when the haemoglobin is less than 7 g/dl (70 g/l). Blue sclera have been described as a sign of iron deficiency anaemia.

Rickets is due to vitamin D deficiency and is manifest by limb pain, widening of wrist bones, knock-knees and the 'rickety rosary'. The 'rickety rosary' is caused by expansion of the costochondral junctions, which are more lateral than many students think.

Clinical signs of rickets include:

- delayed closure of anterior fontanelle
- delayed onset of walking

215

- bow-legged gait, waddling gait
- knock-knees
- expanded painful wrists
- palpable rickety rosary at costochondral junctions
- misery
- relative failure to thrive
- hypotonia, when severe.

Rickets is most often due to dietary vitamin D deficiency plus lack of sunlight in dark-skinned infants living in temperate climates. It is commonly accompanied by signs of anaemia, usually iron deficient.

Protein. Severe protein deficiency is seen in kwashiorkor. The child so affected is apathetic, has flaky skin, reddish thin hair and oedema of the face or legs.

Folic acid, vitamin B$_{12}$ and *vitamin C deficiency* are all rare in Western children. However, scurvy and other vitamin deficiencies may be seen in children fed on strict vegetarian ('vegan') diets.

Obesity is a significant clinical problem, particularly in Western children. Most often this obesity is caused by dietary/environmental/familial factors. Endocrine obesity (secondary to hypothyroidism, Cushing's syndrome, etc.) is by comparison relatively infrequent. Dietary obesity is generalized and usually associated with advanced early growth. Striae may be seen in prepubertal children with rapid weight gain (prepubescent 'puppy fat'). Hormonal and syndromic obesity are usually associated with short stature. The degree of obesity can be gauged by the deviation of the weight centile line from the height centile line, height and weight centiles normally being fairly approximate.

Dietary obesity is generalized (face, arms, legs, trunk and buttocks). Striae at shoulders and hips are frequently seen in prepubertal or adolescent children who gain weight rapidly.

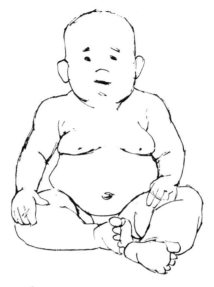

Fig. 7.3 A plump infant.

Body mass index (BMI) is increased, skinfold thickness is increased and blood pressure is often in the upper range of normal.

Anorexia nervosa is most often experienced in adolescent girls. The face is thin, BMI reduced, there is little subcutaneous fat anywhere, arms, thighs and buttocks are thin, thighs don't meet, hips and spine are prominent. Additionally in severe cases the skin may be dry, peripheries cold, pulse relatively slow, and pulse volume reduced. Fine lanugo hair may be seen on face and back. Teeth may be stained as a result of induced vomiting.

8 Developmental assessment

Remember every child is different.

Anon

Developmental assessment is an integral part of paediatric examination and therefore it is essential that normal developmental and normal variations are clearly understood. In general, assessment is ongoing through to adolescence but is of more importance during the preschool period (0–5 years).

Where doubt is raised with respect to development, a detailed perinatal, family and environmental history is essential. Evaluating the child's particular developmental history may be difficult and time consuming – but can be very rewarding and is essential.

A thorough physical examination is essential, particularly looking for minor abnormalities and noting size and shape of head, height and weight. Having established that the child does not have a physical disorder which may influence development, assessment is then based on:

- gross motor status
- vision and fine motor
- hearing and speech
- social behaviour.

Each of these headings is interdependent and complementary. In general terms, an infant's attention span and interest in surroundings is of more importance than gross motor development – particularly if the latter is influenced by obesity or a physical disorder.

The initial age for developmental assessment is 6–8 weeks and is outlined in detail in Chapter 4.

It must be stressed that at any developmental assessment examination both mother and infant should be put at ease and made comfortable. Initial discussion should concern the previous history and enquiry into the general behaviour of the infant to date should be made. Complimentary remarks about infant to mother are helpful. Under no circumstances should one initially attempt physical examination. Sit, watch and observe particularly the size, disposition, appearance and general demeanour of your patient.

3 MONTHS

Gross motor. Holds head erect and steady to 30° and in ventral suspension head is held up for prolonged period. Also can hold shoulders off table when in the prone position.

Vision and fine movement. Appears alert and readily follows objects and has established hand regard. At this stage hands are open and grasp reflex is gone.

Hearing and speech. More responsive to noise and may turn to sound. Babbling is the norm.

4–5 MONTHS

Gross motor. Head control further established, back is straighter.

Vision and fine movement. Regards dangling object and follows – tries to reach with hands. Pulls cloth from face in play. Strabismus must be investigated. Convergence is present.

Hearing. May turn to sound and is very vocal.

6–8 MONTHS: VERY IMPORTANT EXAMINATION

Normal gross motor development at this time will include sitting without support (Fig. 8.1), rolling over and the ability to extend the arms and lift the chest in the prone position. Lateral righting and parachute reflexes are becoming established and sophisticated.

Visual acuity can now be reasonably well assessed. At a distance of 3 m a selection of white balls down to 2 cm will be followed. Eye movement can also be commented on. Strabismus is significant at this age. Improving visual acuity allows for significant development of hand/eye coordination where an infant can reach out and with palmar grasp retrieve a small object (brick) which will be examined, probably transferred to the other hand and finally put to the mouth. Usually hand dominance is not established at this time.

The infant at this age will also turn to sound at a distance of 0.5 m in a horizontal line from the ear. It is often noted that around 5–6 months one ear may respond better than

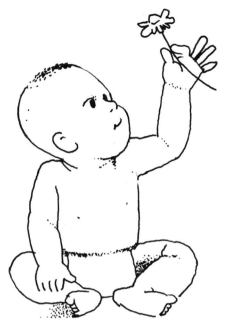

Fig. 8.1 By 6–8 months the infant should be sitting unsupported.

the other. Enhanced response usually occurs in the ear addressed by the nursing mother. The sounds used as stimulus include speech frequencies (500–2000 Hz) with crumpled paper, rattle, and cup and spoon. Socially, the infant is usually happy with strangers, laughs easily, will respond to talking and will be babbling more precisely: that is 'dada', and 'baba'.

Motor:

- good head control
- rolls over
- sits momentarily
- back straight.

Vision and fine movement:

- alert
- eyes move in all directions
- fixates on small object – 20 cm
- palmar grasp – transfers.

Hearing and speech:

- turns to sound 0.5 m
- mother's voice discerned
- vocalizes – 'ka', 'dah'.

Social:

- takes everything to mouth
- tries to hold bottle
- can elicit noise from rattle
- responds to tickling.

Warnings:

- maternal anxiety
- head circumference less than 3rd centile
- hypotonia – poor head control
- hypertonia – brisk reflexes and clonus
- not alert – failure to fixate or strabismus
- not turning to sound (beware unilateral response)
- persistent primitive reflexes.

9–10 MONTHS

Motor:

- sits alone and can turn to look
- can move on floor – rolling, squirming, crawling
- will support weight when upright and will probably hold on
- does not like being moved from sitting to lying supine
- protective reflexes well established.

Vision and fine movement:

- very observant
- pincer grasp with good manipulation (Fig. 8.2)
- looks after fallen toy
- can see small object at 3 m.

Hearing and speech:

- may know and turn to name
- test hearing at 1 m
- babbles loudly and incessantly.

Social:

- holds, bites and chews biscuit
- grasps bottle when feeding
- beginning of suspicion of strangers.

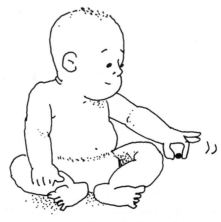

Fig. 8.2 By 9–10 months the infant will demonstrate pincer grasp with good manipulation.

Warnings:

- maternal anxiety
- head circumference < 3rd centile
- not sitting
- poor protective reflexes
- asymmetry of tone
- brisk reflexes or clonus
- poor vocalization
- poor response to sound
- unable to chew.

12 MONTHS

At 12 months there may be considerable variation in developmental status, particularly in gross motor. At this time the infant should be sitting and turning without difficulty. Most will be crawling or have a variation thereof to include rolling over, bottom-shuffling, side-stroking and bear walk (back legs extended). Standing with or without support should be achieved. Some will walk holding on or on their own. In general terms if an infant walks into the examination room aged 1 year, you can almost turn him around and walk him out again.

Visual acuity has improved and a 1-cm diameter ball is followed at 3 m. Objects are now picked up, using the more sophisticated thumb-index finger or pincer grasp. Objects receive more attention and examination. However, they still reach the mouth. The baby will search for an object falling from view. The sound frequencies used for the 5-month-old are now applied at a distance of 1 m from the ear and in a 180° arc at each side. Vocabulary has improved both in pronunciation and number of words (two to three). The infant comprehends simple commands – wave 'day-day', clap hands. Socially the infant is now wary of strangers and clings to his mother. However, he responds to his own name and plays purposefully with toys.

At this age major areas of delay should have surfaced to include – poor brain growth, gross motor delay, visual and hearing impairment and, in particular, cerebral palsy of the spastic type. Even at this early age, prognostic projections are possible.

18 MONTHS

Motor:

- walks
- may run – straight
- creeps backwards downstairs
- picks up toy from floor without falling.

Vision and fine movement:

- builds two to three bricks
- points to distant objects (outside)
- hand preference appearing
- shows distinct interest in human face.

Hearing and language:

- vocalizes freely
- up to 20 words
- plus responds quickly to simple commands.

Social:

- drinks without spilling
- hands cup back to adult
- has stopped putting toys into mouth.

Warnings:

- maternal anxiety
- not standing

- not walking
- poor attention span.

Developmental assessment is an integral part of every clinic visit. We would hope that accurate developmental examination will facilitate early detection of problems. We have itemized early warning signals which make specialized referral mandatory. We would refer you to specialized texts for follow-on examinations at older ages.

Note: The rate of development does vary between children. The sequence of development does not differ significantly. Loss of primitive reflexes is paralleled by a gain of positive skills.

Developmental decisions

- normal
- probably normal – see again
- doubtful – see again soon
- abnormal – refer for diagnosis and treatment

Some commentators prefer the term developmental 'stepping stones' to developmental 'milestones'. Remember that whatever term you use, development is about progress and change. Described below are some locomotion variants to give appreciation of the range of normality.

- Some infants never crawl: they stand and walk.
- Some do normal crawl with flexed knees + some do side-stroke (swing) crawl.
- Some do bear walk (knees extended).
- Some roll from A to B.
- Some bounce around floor or 'bottom-shuffle'.
- Some commando crawl – crawling on elbows rather than hands.

3 YEARS

Can walk up stairs, one foot per step and may be able to jump from bottom step. Stands on one foot momentarily – may be able to ride tricycle.

Builds tower of blocks, can partially dress and will probably draw a circle from a copy. May know one or two colours. There may be three- to five-word sentences and may be able to count to 10. Probably knows full name and can use spoon and fork.

4 YEARS

Assessment of children in this age group is of considerable importance, particularly because of the advent of school. Comprehensive ophthalmological assessment should be carried out at this age. Once again background information in relation to family, siblings, environment and social factors should be carefully checked and analysed.

Gross motor activity has become much more sophisticated to include ability to stand and hop on one foot, can walk downstairs in adult fashion one foot at a time, and can catch a ball, can dress and undress without much help. The use of a pencil to draw objects such as circles, square, a man, with left or right hand now dominant. Now knows three to four colours. Toilet training is well established. Speech has become more sophisticated, talks a lot, asks questions – tells stories.

9 Examining excreta

THE STOOL MEDICAL INSPECTION

Paediatric ward sisters often rightly complain of the lack of interest shown by junior medical staff or students in stools. One wonders how some doctors know what are abnormal stools since they know so little of what is normal. Even when presented suitably wrapped in transparent film and appropriately perfumed, stools are unwillingly examined or observed with haste and distaste.

What is normal stool frequency, consistency, colour, odour? This is determined by feeding contents and pattern. The experienced ward sister knows, of course, that certain conditions can display characteristic stools discernible at a glance. While the descriptions given below are 'classic' examples of certain conditions, recognizable patterns in stool passage and stool appearance amongst infants may direct one down an appropriate diagnostic pathway. When it comes to children's stool medical inspection, listen carefully to the mother's description and the ward sister's interpretation. Also remember that the stools may be apparently 'normal' in proven coeliac or cystic fibrosis.

Breast-fed motions. These are soft, bright yellow (like scrambled eggs) with a fragrant acid odour. Frequency can vary from three to six per day. Volume is usually less than formula motions.

Formula-fed motions are usually more formed than breast-fed stools, will vary from brown to yellowish to a powdery green. Some proprietary formulas do produce characteristic stools.

Hunger stools are now not often seen in Western countries. They are traditionally described as being like spinach, green, loose.

Coeliac disease. The typical stools are large, pale, bulky and offensive. A normal stool pattern, or even constipation, does not exclude coeliac disease.

Cystic fibrosis. The motions are bulky, greasy, and singularly offensive. But are not all stools intrinsically offensive? Certainly. The mother of a child recently diagnosed of cystic fibrosis informed us, 'You'd need a gas mask to change him'.

Toddler diarrhoea (irritable bowel of infancy). The motions are frequent (three to five per day), messy ('they run down his leg, doctor'), brown, mucousy, and contain vegetable matter (especially peas, carrots, corn and tomatoes). The Americans aptly label this 'peas and carrots syndrome'.

Disaccharide intolerance. Frequent, watery, acidic ('they burn his bottom') stools often associated with the passage of flatus.

Acute gastroenteritis. Watery, green, frequent, offensive, poorly formed motions. Bloody diarrhoea may suggest an *Escherichia coli*, *Salmonella* or *Shigella* aetiology. The stools in rotavirus gastroenteritis are said to smell like freshly mown hay. They may contain seed-like material.

Liver disease. Motions may be pale.

Intussusception. Classic motions are described as being 'like redcurrant jelly'. These occur late in intussusception. The important early symptoms are pain, pallor and apparent shock.

Iron. May darken the motions.

Rifampicin. May stain the motions an orange colour.

Worms. Threadworms, roundworms, tapeworms and whipworms may be seen in freshly passed motions.

In conclusion, going through the motions is important in determining the cause of acute and chronic diarrhoeal diseases in children. The start of paediatric gastroenterology is to take oneself to stool examination.

CAST YOUR EYE ON THE URINE

Inspection of sputum, vomitus or stools may be ignored by students (at their peril), but examination of the urine cannot (Fig. 9.1). Urine needs to be inspected, occasionally smelt, 'dipsticked' and subjected to light microscopy. It is beyond the scope of this book to discuss the causes of haematuria, or red urine ('haemastix' negative), or leucocyturia. But we do insist that students know how to interpret routine 'dipstick' analysis for protein, blood, ketones, etc., how to recognize red and white cells on unspun, unstained urine, and how to identify casts. Methods for collecting urine are given in Table 9.1.

On the sideroom door in one London children's unit one used to read the notice: 'Richard Bright omitted to examine the urine with a microscope – you can do better'. (Richard Bright described glomerulonephritis in 1850, but eschewed the microscope.)

Table 9.1 Urine collection

Age	Methods	Comment
Infant	Clean catch	Best; requires patience
Infant	Bladder massage	See page 60
Infant	Bladder percussion	Sometimes works
Infant, toddler	Bag	Remove quickly, avoid contamination
Toddler	Standing in bath	Useful way of getting MSU
Toilet-trained child	Classic MSU	Best
Any	Catheter	Rarely necessary
Infant	Bladder stab	Acutely ill; failed MSU, rarely necessary
Any	Running tap, cold water	Often works!

MSU, midstream urine.

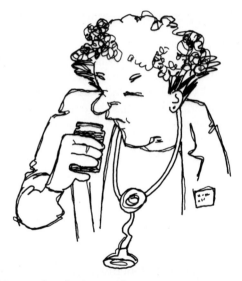

Fig. 9.1 Urine needs to be inspected.

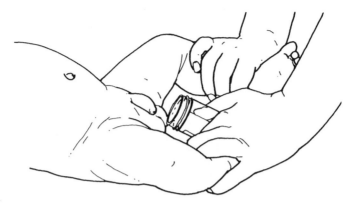

Fig. 9.2 Awaiting a clean catch urine.

Urine colour and concentration can be inspected. Orange urine is induced by jaundice and by rifampicin. The first sign of acute glomerulonephritis may be the passage of red, dark, tea or 'coke'-coloured urine. Dilute watery urine may be seen in diabetes insipidus (central or nephrogenic) and in polydipsic states. The frothiness of albumen-containing urine was first noted in Hippocratic times.

The presence of granular or red cell casts in the urine is pathognomonic of acute glomerulonephritis. Casts should be sought in any child with acute haematuria. With a little tuition and lots of looking students can come to recognize red cells, white cells and bacteria in unstained urine. Time spent peering down the microscope will be repaid in practice. Hyaline casts are a normal finding.

Urine cloudiness is a common finding and may reflect the presence of dissolved chemicals (urates, phosphates) or of leucocytes. Dissolved urates will precipitate out on standing and the sediment frequently has a pinkish hue; this is a normal finding (Table 9.2). The presence of leucocyturia suggests urinary tract infection.

One may occasionally see threadworm cysts in fresh urine.

Urine colours	
red	= haematuria
red (haemastix negative)	= haemoglobinuria, beeturia, phenolphthalein dyes
purple	= porphyria (very rare!)
orange	= jaundice or rifampicin
white	= chyluria
coke-coloured	= glomerulonephritis (usually)
blue	= methylene blue; used to treat methaemoglobinaemia
watery	= polydipsia, either psychogenic or due to diabetes insipidus
pink	= presence of urates
black	= alkaptonuria (very rare)

Table 9.2 Urinalysis

	Probably not infected	Probably infected
Clarity	Clear	Cloudy
Leucocytes	0	+
Blood	0	+
Protein	0	+
Leucostix	−	+

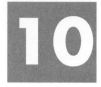

10 Using your senses

A CACOPHONY OF CRIES

> But what am I
> An infant crying in the night
> An infant crying for the light
> And with no language but a cry
>
> Tennyson

Probably the most important, relished and long-awaited cry a child will make in his life is the first exclamatory cry he makes on emerging, relieved, from the birth canal.

The infant's ability to express himself is very limited, especially in his early days and months. The same symptoms – poor feeding, lethargy, vomiting, fever – may signal many different impending infections or illnesses. As such, his cry is of crucial importance as a means of communication. His cry may be trying to tell you something.

235

Mothers soon get to know their baby's collection of 'normal' cries, signifying hunger, wind, wet, dirty or loneliness. Students, too, need to open their ears and listen (Fig. 10.1).

A short period of nursing duties – feeding, changing, observing babies – is of considerable value to all students during their paediatric course. It cannot be said too often – you will not readily recognize the abnormal unless you are familiar with the normal.

We wish to refer briefly to:

- cries of pain
- cries of certain illnesses
- cries of some conditions.

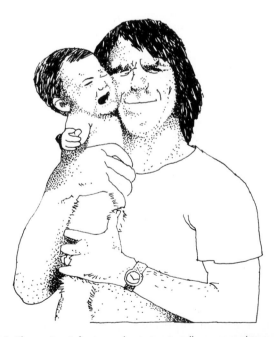

Fig. 10.1 The crying infant may be trying to tell you something.

Painful cries

Probably the most important cry to recognize is that of pain in infancy. The most alarming cry is that heard in association with meningitis, encephalitis, or raised intra-cranial pressure from whatever cause. Mothers will usually describe this as high-pitched, shrill, screeching, screaming or piercing (Fig. 10.2). Always take note of the mother who says, 'His cry has changed, it's different'. In addition to the particular cry, infants with intracranial lesions can be diffi-cult to console. The cry which accompanies infantile spasms can be short, sharp, high-pitched and is not infrequently thought to be due to 'colic'. It is not unusual for a cry to accompany an epileptic seizure.

In short, the cry of pain is different from the infant's usual cry and mother will usually detect this call. So listen to her.

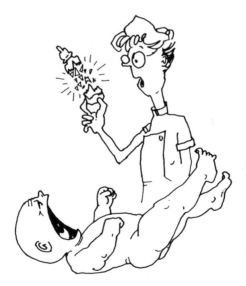

Fig. 10.2 Infant cry.

Cries of illness

The cry of acute croup is hoarse. The cough in croup resembles the bark of a seal (sea lion). The cry of acute bronchopneumonia may be weak and grunting. The cry of the infant with acute intussusception may be sudden and grunting. The severely ill infant has a weak, whimpering cry.

Characteristic cries

Characteristic cries are described in certain conditions. Congenital hypothyroidism (hopefully soon an obsolete condition with extension of screening) is associated with a hoarse, croaky cry. Once heard, the extraordinary mewling of the cri-du-chat syndrome is never forgotten. Crowing cry may indicate laryngomalacia or other laryngeal lesion.

All babies cry. It is normal to cry. Don't forget the baby who 'never cries' – he is not normal; one might suspect developmental delay with such a description.

A SENSE OF DIAGNOSIS

Most of us are well trained in using our eyes, hands and ears in aiding diagnosis but often unskilled in the remaining two senses, those of taste and smell. Some brief examples:

- phenylketonuria – 'mousy' smell from urine
- diabetic ketoacidosis – acetone on breath
- maple syrup urine disease – smell of fresh maple sap from urine
- fishy urine – ? *Proteus* infection
- salty taste on kissing – may suggest cystic fibrosis.

THE DIAGNOSTIC TOUCH

At various parts of this text we have emphasized the importance of inspection and palpation in paediatric physical examination.

Teach the back of or ulnar border of your hand to detect changes in temperature. Always palpate rashes (see p. 147). Allow your finger pulps the experience of palpating little pulses in head, hands and feet of infants.

THE LAST WORD

This text will have failed in its primary objectives if students merely read it and fail to apply the principles. It is very difficult to learn how to drive a car or to operate a computer from the manual. So go to it, and examine as many children as will allow you!

11 Paediatric tips and topics

NORMAL FINDINGS

- Telangiectasia (spider naevi) on hands or face of children. One to three telangiectasia is a frequent finding in schoolchildren.
- Café-au-lait spots – a few scattered. More than six larger than 1.5 cm in diameter is suggestive of neurofibromatosis.
- Lymph nodes – scattered small, shotty nodes (see p. 131).
- Innocent (physiological flow) murmurs. Very common.
- Stork-beak marks (capillary haemangiomas) on forehead and nape of neck.
- Epstein's (epithelial) pearls on roof of mouth.
- Slight breast swelling in male and female infants.
- Sacrococcygeal pits and dimples.
- Mongolian blue spots in African/Asian infants and in infants of mixed parentage.
- Sinus arrhythmia.
- Periodic breathing (in premature neonates but *not* in infancy).
- Acrocyanosis (peripheral cyanosis) in newborn.
- Forehead bruises on toddlers who have recently acquired the skill of walking.
- Mild bow-leggedness in toddlers.
- Bruises (as many as 10–20) on knees and shins of active toddlers and preschool children.
- Blue sclerae in infants.
- Single transverse palmar crease – in up to 5% of children.

TOOLS OF THE TRADE

1. Stethoscope, preferably with 'paediatric' bell and diaphragm.
2. Tape measure, preferably steel or disposable. Plastic tapes may stretch if boiled.
3. Appropriate centile charts for boys and girls of different ages.
4. Sphygmomanometer – with a selection of cuff widths.

5. Auriscope with earpieces of varying size. Use the largest ear piece which fits comfortably. A piece of rubber tubing to apply suction may be useful.
6. A good light source for examining the fauces.
7. An ophthalmoscope. Remember that children dislike bright lights shone in their eyes. Keep light intensity down.
8. A pencil and paper – to allow the child to write or draw when you're talking to his mother.
9. A selection of picture and reading books (for example in the 'Ladybird' series).
10. A few toys.
11. Some bricks.
12. A mirror.
13. A rattle.
14. A bell.
15. Magnifying glass for looking at skin lesions.

Plus (if possible) 'the same kind, beaming smile that children could warm their hands at' (JM Barrie)

Some departments of child health will have simulators, on which useful experience and practice may be obtained without distressing or harming anyone. Some examples:

1. Baby Hippy, Medical Plastics, Chicago.
2. Resusci Baby, Laerdal, Norway.
3. Ophthalmoscopy mannequin, Ophthalmic Development Lab., Iowa, USA.

TRICKS OF THE TRADE

1. Listening over the nose with a stethoscope (see p. 136).
2. Distraction techniques (see pp. 37–38).
3. Use of the thumbs to palpate pulses is permissible (if not desirable). Some may better be able to fix and palpate femoral pulses of the wriggling infant with the thumbs than with the finger pulps.

4. Palpating over the child's hands in assessing abdominal pain or tenderness (see p. 43).
5. Use of the stethoscope to gauge doubtful abdominal 'tenderness' (see pp. 42, 44).
6. The auriscope is best held in a penhold grip – you are less likely to hurt the child (see pp. 134, 135).
7. Use of auriscope to look up noses (for foreign bodies).
8. To get a newborn infant to open his eyes, hold him upright, or give him something to suck (see p. 192) Don't try to prise the eyes open – it just doesn't work.
9. When assessing plagiocephaly (parallelogram skull), place a finger in each auditory canal and compare their relative positions (see pp. 54–55).
10. Asking children to point to the site of the pain (see pp. 41, 42)
11. When looking at the throat ask the child to make a big yawn (see p. 137).
12. Keep preschool and playschool children on their feet for as much of the examination as possible – they feel much less threatened.
13. Flatter children on how good they are, on a nice dress or shirt, or tell him he's the boss in his family.
14. Strike up a rapport by talking at child level or discussing his favourite television show (e.g. *Teletubbies*).
15. If in doubt about undescended testes, examine the child while he is squatting (see pp. 124, 125)

BIOLOGICAL WARNING SIGNS

- The infant who loves (and licks) salt – has he a salt-losing state, for example cystic fibrosis or a tubulopathy?
- The toddler who throws away bread and biscuits. Could this suggest coeliac disease?
- The child who hates soft drinks and sweets. Should you consider sucrase-isomaltase deficiency?

- The child who drinks *anything* – he may have true diabetes insipidus. In addition, he will usually wake at night seeking drinks.
- The child who objects to milk – give lactose intolerance or milk allergy a thought.
- The child who lies down. He is ill. Sick children are like animals – they lie down when ill (without having to be told to do so) and get up when better.
- Refusal or unwillingness to move a limb usually suggests something serious – a fracture or osteomyelitis, for example.
- Children with chronic renal insufficiency usually have a preference for water rather than milk or sweet drinks.
- The child who eats well but nevertheless fails to thrive. Consider a malabsorption state such as cystic fibrosis.
- The child for whom exercise of any sort results in coughing or shortness of breath. This is almost diagnostic of bronchial asthma.

CLINICAL CURIOS

1. *The allergic salute*. Children with allergic rhinitis frequently rub their nose vigorously with the palm of their hand.
2. *'Screwdriving'*. Agitated or upset infants have a characteristic habit of rotating their hands in a screwdriving motion.
3. *Yawning*. In the newborn may be indicative of seizure activity.
4. *'Cracked pot note'* is the sound obtained on percussing the skull in infants with raised intracranial pressure.
5. *Foreign bodies* may end up in nostrils, ears, vaginas, as well as in stomachs and chests.
6. We have come to respect two symptoms in infants and toddlers – *limp and torticollis*. Whereas a limp has many causes, a lingering limp is a well-recognized presentation of acute leukaemia. Acute head tilt is unusual in early

245

childhood – consider posterior fossa tumour in the absence of other explanation.

7. Most *breath-holding episodes* terminate spontaneously. Some may, however, progress to 'pallid syncope' (a vasovagal episode) or even to 'reflex anoxic seizures'.

8. Lip-smacking and cycling lower limb movements are involuntary in the first 48 hours of life and are associated with asphyxial encephalopathy.

9. Sandifer's syndrome: arching, posturing, apparent dystonic movements which occur in children with reflux oesophagitis. The movements occur after eating and may be thought to be convulsions.

10. How would you recognize the adult who was breast-fed? Feel the tip of his nose. In sucklings, the physical effects of breast pressure result in the two nasal cartilages being kept separate. In bottle-fed children the nasal cartilages unite and present in the adult as a single sharp outline.

11. Chronically ill children have long lush eyelashes.

RULES OF THUMB

- All that wheezes is not asthma, but when recurrent usually is.
- All that whoops is not pertussis, but most is. Adenovirus and parapertussis may produce a whoop.
- The more widespread the pain, the less likely it is to be organic.
- An infant who continues to feed may be ill, but not seriously so.
- Viral infections tend to spread (ears, throat, skin, e.g. measles), whereas bacterial infections tend to localize (one ear, lobe of lung, pointing abscess) – Lightwood's law.
- The primary duty of any hospital children's doctor is to discharge children therefrom.
- Mother is right until proved otherwise.
- One of the primary functions of tonsils is to get infected.

- Inspection might better be considered as observation.
- If you find one major malformation look for others: malformations tend to be multiple.
- Students should not be systems specialists.
- Really sick children do not smile.
- Seriously ill children lie absolutely still.
- Cold extremities are a sign of serious illness, perhaps impending hypovolaemic shock.

MATERNAL MYTHS

While we are continually impressed by the correctness of maternal instincts, there are certain myths that mothers persist in perpetrating. Below are some examples that students may meet – try compiling your own list from your clients.

1. Nose picking is associated with intestinal worms.
2. Laxatives will 'clear badness out of children'.
3. Strapping, strictures and mercurochrome will cure thumb-sucking.
4. Worms are a cause of bed wetting (rarely true).
5. A copper penny will cure umbilical hernias (they resolve themselves).
6. Goat's milk is good for eczema.
7. Breast-fed babies are never obese (ask a student of medieval art – chubby cherubs abound).
8. Caries in primary teeth doesn't matter ('sweet tooths' carry on!).
9. Teething causes convulsions (teething produces teeth).
10. Early walking produces bow legs.
11. Orange pips lodge in the appendix.

ACRIMONIOUS ACRONYMS

TORCH = toxoplasmosis, other, rubella, cytomegalovirus, herpes
NTD   = neural tube defect

CDH   = congenital dislocated hips
CHD   = congenital heart disease
FLK   = 'funny looking kid'; a term best avoided
IRDS   = idiopathic respiratory distress syndrome
LBW   = low birth weight
VLBW   = very low birth weight
SGA   = small for gestational age (sometimes called 'light for
         dates', 'small for dates')
IDM   = infant of diabetic mother
IVH   = intraventricular haemorrhage
CPAP   = continuous positive airways pressure
PEEP   = positive end-expiratory pressure
IPPV   = intermittent positive pressure ventilation
NEC   = necrotizing enterocolitis
PFC   = persistent fetal circulation
BPD   = bronchopulmonary dysplasia
RLF   = retrolental fibroplasia
TTN   = transient tachypnoea of newborn
TAPVD = total anomalous pulmonary venous drainage
ZIG   = zoster immune globulin
DTP   = diphtheria, tetanus, pertussis (also called 'triple
         antigen')
FAS   = fetal alcohol syndrome.

We all use acronyms. Don't pepper your notes or your examination paper with too many of them. Remember that MI can stand for myocardial infarct, mitral incompetence, mental illness or a well-known motorway.

A–Z OF EPONYMS

Alport's syndrome	= congenital nephritis plus deafness
Apert's syndrome	= acrocephaly plus syndactyly
Arnold–Chiari malformation	= displacement of medulla and cerebellum into spinal canal

Barlow's manoeuvre	= technique of examining for congenitally dislocated hips
Barr bodies	= chromatin mass in cell nuclei
Beckwith–Wiedemann syndrome	= enlarged tongue, enlarged viscera, gigantism
Berger's disease	= IgA nephropathy
Bright's disease (obsolete)	= post-streptococcal glomerulonephritis
Blackfan–Diamond syndrome	= congenital pure red cell aplasia
Caffey's disease	= infantile cortical hyperostosis
Cornelia de Lange's syndrome	= mental and physical retardation, typical facies
Crigler–Najjar syndrome	= rare deficiency of glucuronyl transferase
Dandy–Walker malformation	= atresia of foramina of Magendie and Luschka
Di George syndrome	= congenital aplasia of the thymus
Duckett–Jones criteria	= criteria for diagnosis of rheumatic fever
Epstein's pearls	= epithelial pearls on roof of mouth
Erb's palsy	= upper arm type of brachial palsy
Fallot's tetralogy	= ventricular septal defect, pulmonary stenosis, right ventricular hypertrophy, over-riding aorta
Fanconi's anaemia	= congenital aplastic anaemia
Fanconi's syndrome (also known as de Toni–Debré–Fanconi syndrome)	= phospho-gluco-amino acid bicarbonaturia, proximal tubular leak
Gilbert's syndrome	= persistent unconjugated hyperbilirubinaemia

Guillain–Barré syndrome = ascending polyneuritis

Hand–Schüller–Christian disease = a form of histiocytosis with diabetes insipidus and bone lesions

Henoch–Schönlein syndrome = vasculitis, arthritis, nephritis, abdominal pain

Hirschsprung's disease = colonic aganglionosis

Kaposi's varicelliform eruption = herpetic skin lesions in eczematous children

Kawasaki's disease = mucocutaneous lymph node syndrome

Klinefelter's syndrome = phenotype associated with XXY genotype

Koplik's spots = white spots on buccal mucosa in measles prodrome

Laurence–Moon–Biedl syndrome = polydactyly, obesity, mental retardation

Louis–Bar syndrome = ataxia telangiectasia

Lowe's syndrome = oculocerebrorenal syndrome

Marfan's syndrome = dislocated lens, tall stature, weak aortic wall

Meckel's diverticulum = aberrant ectopic gastric mucosa

Morgan–Dennie fold = double infraorbital fold in eczematous children

Noonan's syndrome = XO phenotype in the male, pulmonary stenosis

Ortolani's test = for congenital hip dislocation

Potter's facies = squashed newborn facies associated with oligohydramnios

Reye's syndrome = acute encephalopathy and liver failure

Ritter's disease = scalded skin syndrome

Russell–Silver syndrome	= triangular facies, short stature, body asymmetry
Sprengel's deformity	= congenital upward displacement of the scapula
Treacher Collins syndrome	= mandibulofacial dysostosis
von Gierke's disease (obsolete)	= glycogen storage disease
von Recklinghausen's disease (obsolete)	= neurofibromatosis
von Willebrand's disease (obsolescent)	= factor VIII deficiency
Wilms' tumour	= nephroblastoma
Zellweger's syndrome	= cerebrohepatorenal syndrome.

The above list is by no means exhaustive. Eponyms are abused entities and should be discarded when the true nature of the described entity or syndrome becomes clear. Happily we have ended our list with examples of obsolete or obsolescent eponyms. Much as we would all like to have a memorable eponymous syndrome, so-named children benefit when the syndrome is untangled and its components elucidated. Do remember that what today's doctors label as, for example, Henoch–Schönlein syndrome, may not resemble what the good German doctors described a century ago.

There is a certain mystique about nobly named syndromes and doctors which failed to impress Matthew Arnold who wrote as follows:

> Nor bring to watch me cease to live,
> Some doctor full of phrase and fame,
> To shake his sapient head and give
> The ill man can not cure – a name.

Eponymic syndromes might be described as a baptized collection of signs and symptoms awaiting confirmation.

Dublin has abandoned Graves' disease in favour of thyrotoxicosis, Guy's Hospital has allowed glomerulonephritis to supplant Bright's disease and Corrigan's pulse has irrevocably collapsed.

ALARM SIGNALS: ? NON-ACCIDENTAL INJURIES

Listed below is a selection of physical signs which may be suggestive of inflicted rather than accidental injuries:

- torn frenulum in bottle-fed infants
- black eyes in toddlers
- finger marks on cheeks
- petechiae on the pinna
- scratch marks
- teeth imprints anywhere
- punched-out burns (cigarettes?)
- bruises in non-traumatic sites
- retinal haemorrhages
- perivaginal bruises
- bruises of varying ages.

In addition, the experienced observer may recognize as being alerting:

- 'frozen watchfulness' (a cold unemotional look)
- persistent gaze avoidance
- extremely unkempt appearance
- severe nappy rash.

Proper notekeeping is imperative in non-accidental injury. The marks, bruises or injuries must be described, drawn and, if possible, photographed. The accumulated evidence will be very important in the subsequent case conference and any court proceedings which may ensue. Efforts to age bruises or injuries require considerable experience and clinical expertise.

MEMORABLE MNEMONICS

There are many memorable mnemonics in medicine. They are often passed on by students from generation to generation. Some collect and retain mnemonics, others abhor them. Some students compose their own. If our memories serve us right, memorable mnemonics can be useful in the stress of examinations.

Here are a few simple examples. Some are old favourites, some have been suggested by our students, and some are our own creations. We would appreciate good examples from other sources.

1. *Triggers of childhood asthma = ASTHMA*
   A = allergy (house dust mite, pollens, dander)
   S = sport (exercise, play)
   T = temperature (cold, wet, windy weather)
   H = heredity (familial tendency to asthma; gene locus)
   M = microbiology (viruses, mycoplasma, etc.)
   A = anxiety (stress, worries).
2. *Assessing severity of asthma – 6 Ss*
   School – how much missed?
   Sleep – how much disturbance?
   Sport – how able? opting out?
   Social activities – how much disruption?
   Symptom score card – how severe?
   Steroids – drug requirements?
3. *6 Is of eczema*
   I for itch (antihistamines, etc.)
   I for ichthyosis (emollients, etc.)
   I for inflammation (topical steroids)
   I for infection (antibiotics)
   I for irritability (because of above)
   I for self-image (psychological support)
4. *5 Ds for epiglottitis (supraglottitis)*
   Drooling

Dysphagia
Dysphonia
Dyspnoea
Distress
A final, dreaded, but possible 'D' in epiglottitis is death.

5. *Causes of splenomegaly = SPLEEN*
   Sequestration (of RBCs in haemolytic anaemias)
   Proliferation (viral infections, etc.)
   Lipid accumulation (Gaucher's, etc.)
   Engorgement (portal hypertension)
   Endowment (haemangiomas, cysts)
   INvasion (malignancies).

6. *Rheumatic fever has a number of fives*
   5 major criteria:
   carditis
   arthritis
   chorea
   subcutaneous nodules
   erythema marginatum
   5 minor criteria:
   prolonged PR interval
   past history of rheumatic fever
   arthralgia
   positive laboratory tests (erythrocyte sedimentation rate
   (ESR), anti-streptolysin titre (ASO), etc.)
   pyrexia

Affects age 5–15 years primarily. Commoner below 50°N and 50°S latitude. At least 5 years' prophylaxis for carditis.

7. *PS = Pyloric stenosis*
   PV = projectile vomiting
   PV = peristalsis visible
   PT = palpable tumour
   PS = positive scan (ultrasound)
   PR = pyloromyotomy Ramstedt

8. *Why circumcisions are performed: 6 Ms*
   Moses (Jewish religion)
   Mohammed (Muslims)
   Mother wants it
   Money
   Mythical reasons
   Medical reasons (phimosis, paraphimosis)
9. *ABC of haematuria*
   Anatomy (cysts, etc.)
   Bladder (cystitis)
   Cancer (Wilms' tumour)
   Drug-related (cyclophosphamide)
   Exercise induced
   Factitious (Munchausen by proxy)
   Glomerulonephritis (casts+)
   Haematology (bleeding disorder, sickle cell)
   Infection (urinary tract infection (UTI))
   In**J**ury (trauma)
   Kidney stones (hypercalciuria)
   In reality and in rank the main causes in children are:
   Infection (UTI)
   Inflammation (glomerulonephritis)
   Injury (trauma)
   Hypercalciuria and calculi

The other causes are relatively rare. Age, presence or absence of pain, and urinary symptoms are other relevant factors.

10. *The three most important Ps in paediatrics are, in our opinion*:
    Parenting
    Poverty
    Prevention
11. *5As of EBM (evidence-based medicine)*
    Ask the question
    Access the information

Appraise the evidence
Apply the answers
Assess the process
12. *Bloody diarrhoea = CESSY*
Campylobacter
E. coli
Salmonella
Shigella
Yersinia

While most intellectual academics disparage rote learning, they probably all practised it as students. We would suggest that composition of mnemonics can be fun, and if reliably absorbed, may be recalled at moments when quick thinking is required.

GENETIC GRAPHICS (Fig. 11.1)

A good family tree, well drawn, is the key to genetic mapping. The figure shows two basic pedigrees for a recessive and a dominant condition. Please refer to your paediatric text or to a genetics book for a more detailed exposition and discussion. A well-drawn pedigree will enhance the notes and will be much more visible and more available than a written version. We encourage you to draw family trees as part of your routine history taking.

'GROWING OUT' OF DISORDERS/ILLNESSES

One of the pleasures of paediatrics is that children tend to get better, both in spite of and in response to doctors and medications. Often, the doctor's job is to help children and parents cope with and control illnesses while nature cures. You will experience many such conditions during your paediatric course. Below are some examples:

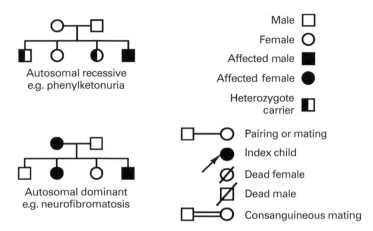

Male ☐
Female ○
Affected male ■
Affected female ●
Heterozygote carrier ◧

Pairing or mating
Index child
Dead female
Dead male
Consanguineous mating

Fig. 11.1 Two examples of family trees.

- asthma
- eczema
- enuresis (about 15% remit annually from age 5 years)
- constitutional short stature
- lactose intolerance
- idiopathic epilepsy
- minimal change variety of nephrotic syndrome
- gastro-oesophageal reflux
- mild-moderate vesico-ureteric reflux
- toddler diarrhoea ('peas and carrots syndrome')
- small ventricular septal defects.

Feel free to add to this list. Contributions for further editions of this text are always welcome. Would the question: 'Write an essay on childhood conditions which have a tendency to remit spontaneously with time' be a fair one? For deeper thinkers, what are the physiological mechanisms governing spontaneous remission of asthma, epilepsy, nephrotic syndrome, et al.?

'THE CHILD IS FATHER OF THE MAN'

William Wordsworth (1770–1850)

There is increasing evidence and acceptance of the fact that many types of adult ill health have their genesis in childhood. Many of the factors implicated in essential hypertension – salt intake, cholesterol, obesity, stress, body weight, physical fitness – accumulate from childhood and adolescence. This notion is not a new one as the following quotations will demonstrate.

We dig our graves with our teeth.

There are only four stages of man – infancy, childhood, adolescence and obsolescence.

Anon

The childhood shows the man, As morning shows the day.

John Milton (1608–1674)

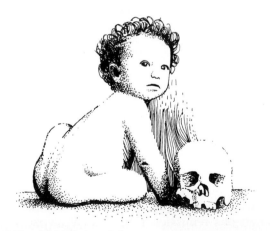

Fig. 11.2 The child is father of the man.

Adults are obsolete children.

Dr Seuss (1904–1991)

What is an adult? A child blown up by age.

Simone de Beauvoir

It is not easy to straighten in the oak the crook that grew in the sapling.

Gaelic proverb

A man is as old as his arteries.

Thomas Sydenham (17th century)

The fate of countries depends on the way they feed themselves.

Anthelme Brillat-Saverin (18th century)

I hardly know whether any argument is necessary to prove that the future of a country must, under God, be laid in the character and condition of its children . . . as the sapling has been bent, so it will grow.

Lord Shaftesbury (1870)

Give a little love to a child, and you get a great deal back.

John Ruskin

Men are but children of a larger growth.

John Dryden

TIPS FOR THE PAEDIATRIC EXAMINATION

Assessment in paediatrics now usually consists of in-course (continuous) assessment and end-of-course examination. It may include case studies, project presentation, written paper, multiple choice questionnaire, objective structured clinical examination and oral.

The following remarks refer to the more traditional type of examination with a prepared long case, and one or more short, unprepared cases. The examiners want to know if you are competent and confident in handling children. They do not seek omniscience – if you don't know the answer to something, say so, rather than hazarding guesses.

Some simple commonsense rules to remember:

1. Extract from the mother or guardian all the information you can obtain. Remember that children with chronic conditions (heart disease, cystic fibrosis) can be remarkably informative. Don't give the child food or sweets without first checking with sister or staff nurse.

2. Observe the child for the first few minutes before making physical contact. Note any observable clinical signs related to symptoms in the history. Assess the degree of illness (well, ill, quite ill). Comment on developmental status (alertness, social interaction, etc.).

3. Above all, be gentle with the child despite your apprehension.

4. Don't forget to weigh and measure the child and plot on appropriate centile charts.

5. Perform a thorough systematic examination, leaving possibly unpleasant bits to the end.

6. Present the relevant positive historical factors first. Try to put the positive clinical findings in order of their importance. If you have come to a conclusion with which you are comfortable say so: 'This is Johnny Murphy, aged 5 years, who has features of Down's syndrome, has a murmur compatible with a ventricular septal defect, and has an abdominal scar consistent with repaired duodenal atresia'.

7. Suggest a differential diagnosis on the basis of positive clinical findings. If pressed for a possible diagnosis always 'back the favourite' and go for common conditions, avoiding rare conditions ('outside chances') unless very sure of them.

8. Don't make your examiners work unnecessarily – try to lead the discussion. If given the opportunity to reconsider your

findings, be sure to avail of it. Examiners are usually trying to help, not to trip.

9. Relax, relax if possible. Your examiners are seeking confidence and competence. If you are well trained, you should have both attributes.

10. Above all, please don't guess, don't fabricate, if you don't know something. Better by far to admit, 'I'm afraid I don't know'.

Objective structured clinical examination (OSCE)

Space does not permit detailed advice. However, the same basic rules as in short cases prevail:

- look at, observe, and note what is being asked
- study the rash, growth chart, referral letter, radiograph or whatever is being presented to you
- think logically before you talk
- time is of the essence, so don't deliberately waste time.

Sample OSCE stations will include urinalysis, demonstration of inhaler technique, recognition of rashes, analysis of biochemical results, etc.

ESSENTIAL CLINICAL SKILLS

We have drawn up this list for our own undergraduate students. We hope that they will use it as a checklist during their paediatric clinical course. While there may be some disagreement about individual items on our list, we think that most paediatric departments will agree with its overall tenor and content. Students need to distinguish between things that they 'need to know' versus items that are 'nice to know'.

We hope that this list is helpful and not off-putting. We suspect that it is much shorter and less daunting than the checklist of quality control tests applied to any new car rolling off the automobile assembly line. Entry requirements to medical school are high. We believe that paediatric skills at exit should be equally high. Hopefully well-trained and well-tuned students will enhance their skills and improve their expertise throughout their working lives.

Essential clinical skills for undergraduate students

Ability to take full history from parents and child.
Ability to perform thorough clinical examination on infant, toddler, older child.
Recognition of the wide range of normality.
Ability to draw conclusions from history and examination with a view to differential diagnosis, planned investigation and therapeutic options.

1. *Cardiovascular system*

☐ Measurement of blood pressure.
☐ Palpation of heart and major arteries.
☐ Detection of right and left ventricular enlargement.
☐ Palpation of thrill.
☐ Auscultation of heart sounds, including added sounds.
☐ Detection and description of significant cardiac murmurs.
☐ Detection of cyanosis, clubbing, polycythaemia.
☐ Demonstration of features of congestive heart failure.
☐ Recognition of innocent flow murmurs.

2. *Respiratory system*

☐ Inspection for signs of respiratory distress.
☐ Percussion of chest.
☐ Appreciation of chest deformities.
☐ Auscultation of normal and adventitious chest sounds.

☐ Ability to detect and describe significant collapse/ consolidation, pleural effusion, pneumothorax.

3. *Abdomen*

☐ Palpation for liver, spleen.
☐ Percussion of liver margins.
☐ Detection of abdominal masses.
☐ Demonstration of ascites.
☐ Differentiation between abdominal swelling due to flatus, fluid, faeces.
☐ Appreciation of normal penile and testicular appearances in boys.
☐ Examination for hydrocele, hernia, undescended testes.
☐ Palpation and percussion of enlarged full bladder.

4. *Skin*

☐ Recognition of common birthmarks, including haemangiomas, naevi, etc.
☐ Recognition and description of rashes of eczema, psoriasis, impetigo, purpura.
☐ Recognition of the exanthema of common infectious diseases, including measles, rubella, chickenpox, scarlet fever.
☐ Detection of jaundice at various sites.
☐ Recognition of vitiligo, café-au-lait spots.
☐ Demonstration of signs of moderate and severe dehydration.

5. *Joints*

☐ Ability to test range of movement in major joints – wrist, elbow, shoulder, hip, knee, ankle. Active and passive movements.
☐ Ability to detect signs of joint inflammation – redness, heat, pain, swelling and loss of function.

6. Neurological

- ☐ Use of reflex hammer to demonstrate deep tendon reflexes.
- ☐ Ability to test for meningism.
- ☐ Appreciation of normal and abnormal fontanelle size and tension.
- ☐ Assessment of tone, gait, coordination, sensation.
- ☐ Visual fields.
- ☐ Detection of variations in muscle tone.
- ☐ Appreciation of major types of cerebral palsy.

7. Measurement

- ☐ Length and height.
- ☐ Weight.
- ☐ Head circumference.
- ☐ Plotting on appropriate centile chart.
- ☐ Puberty staging.

8. Development

- ☐ Assessment at 6 weeks.
- ☐ Assessment at 6 months.
- ☐ Assessment at 1 year.
- ☐ Demonstration of primitive reflexes – Moro, grasp, sucking, tonic, neck, etc.
- ☐ Assessment of hearing and vision at 6 months.
- ☐ Appreciation of gross deviation from normal development.

9. Congenital abnormality

- ☐ Recognition of major syndromes, especially Down's syndrome.
- ☐ Recognition of major malformation, such as myelomeningocele and hydrocephalus.

10. General

☐ Recognition of acute severe illness.
☐ Assessment of nutrition, especially undernutrition and obesity.
☐ Determination of normal hydration.
☐ Detection of anaemia.
☐ Inspection of teeth and gums for evidence of caries and gingival disease.
☐ Recognition of types of cleft lip and palate.

11. Orthopaedics

☐ Testing for congenital dislocation of hip.
☐ Examination of the back for scoliosis.
☐ Trendelenburg's test.
☐ Ability to measure lower limbs for true and apparent shortening.

12. Ear, nose and throat

☐ Use of auriscope.
☐ Examination of fauces and throat.
☐ Weber's and Rinne's tests.

13. Ophthalmology

☐ Examination of external eye.
☐ Testing pupil reactions.
☐ Assessment of eye movements.
☐ Performance of cover test.
☐ Ophthalmoscopy.

THINGS TO BE SEEN AND UNDERSTOOD BY UNDERGRADUATE STUDENTS

The good learner is the active, involved, self-motivated student, who is around the wards, present in the accident and emergency department and willing to assist or observe in theatre. The list below is for guidance only, recognizing that paediatric units/hospitals will involve undergraduate students to varying degrees.

A. Must see:

- lumbar puncture
- bladder catheterization
- insertion of intravenous line
- immunization
- urine collection in infancy
- passage of nasogastric tube.

B. Good to see:

- fluid resuscitation
- endotracheal intubation
- management of diabetic ketoacidosis
- skin scraping for meningococcal sepsis
- intraosseous infusion
- cardiopulmonary resuscitation
- 'Heel prick' test (Guthrie's test)
- electroencephalography
- ultrasonography
- appendicectomy
- air reduction of intussusception
- sweat test.

C. Participate if possible/permissible:

- child abuse case conference
- paediatric post-mortem
- multidisciplinary team meeting.

CLINIQUIZ

1. Describe the features of finger clubbing. What are its causes in childhood?
2. What is sinus arrhythmia?
3. List six skills acquired by a 12-month-old infant.
4. Describe the rash of atopic eczema.
5. What are the features of an innocent/physiological/flow murmur?
6. Give four explanations for a large head in infancy.
7. What are (a) chorea, (b) cogwheel rigidity, (c) anasarca?
8. Clinically how might you distinguish laryngotracheobronchitis from epiglottitis?
9. What did (a) Kernig, (b) Koplik, (c) Korotkoff describe?
10. What is the physiology of squatting in cyanotic heart disease?
11. Why do babies with respiratory difficulty grunt?
12. What are (a) pulsus paradoxus, (b) pulsus alternans, (c) collapsing pulse?
13. Why do infants become mottled when ill?
14. What is the purpose of shivering?
15. Think of five explanations for an acute limp in a 3-year-old child.
16. List five causes of meningism other than meningitis.
17. Which is the diastolic pressure point – phase 4 (muffling) or phase 5 (disappearance of sounds)?
18. Give four causes of acute wheezing in infants.
19. List 10 patterns of injury suggestive of non-accidental injury.
20. Name some drugs which may be associated with hirsutism.
21. The average 2-year-old child is one-third, one-half or two-thirds of his adult height?
22. Is a single transverse palmar crease a normal finding?
23. Most children whose height falls below the third centile lines are 'small normal children'. True or false?

24. How would you distinguish true polydipsia from habit (compulsive, psychogenic) polydipsia in a preschool child?
25. Children's peak expiratory flow rate best correlates with age, sex, height or chest expansion?
26. Blood pressure tends to rise throughout life. Is this 'normal'?
27. What is a bull neck?
28. What is a buffalo hump?
29. Whose cough resembles that of a sea lion?
30. What are wormian bones?

We have resisted providing answers for this cliniquiz, preferring students to seek the answers for themselves.

CHILDREN'S 'WISDOMISMS'

Children can sometimes be startlingly wise in their sayings, combining a simplicity of thought and of expression. Below are cited a few examples from our outpatients and from the collections of Nanette Newman.

(If only breast milk came in a packet?)

When you are a baby your mother feeds you from her bosom, but she can only do milk.

Girl aged 7

(A very modern little lady?)

When I grow up, I will have lots of babies. Then I'll get married and live happily ever after.

Girl aged 6

(A good description of hypoglycaemia by a small boy.)

I get dizzy in my legs.

Boy aged 5

(Abdominal migraine.)

I get a headache in my tummy.

Boy aged 9

An ulcer is like a laser beam going through your stomach.

Boy aged 11

My mother only likes babies. When they get older, like me, she smacks them.

Girl aged 8

Babies need to be loved by their mother in case everybody hates them when they grow up.

Boy aged 7

(Explaining her paraplegia.)

I was born in a wheelchair.

Girl aged 9

PAEDIATRIC SYNONYMS AND SLANG

This short collection is offered for readers whose first language is not English and who may be confused by the meaning of the words and by differing English/American slang.

Synonyms	Slang
Abdomen	tummy, belly
Anus	back passage
Bottom, buttock	bum, butt
Bow-legged, genu varus	bandy
Clavicle	collarbone
Constipation	bunged up
Diaper	nappy
Faeces, stool, bowel motion	poo, etc.
Feverish, febrile	'boiling'
Genitalia	private parts
Infusion, IV	drip
Pacifier, soother, teat	dummy

Penis	willie, wee-man, etc.
Ptosis	droopy
Seizure, convulsion	fit
Sternum	breastbone
Strabismus	crooked eye, squint, turn
Talipes	club foot
Testis, testicles	balls
Torticollis	wry neck
Trachea	windpipe
Umbilicus, navel	belly button
Urine	pee, piss, wee, piddle
Vomiting, puking	throwing up

CHILDREN ARE DIFFERENT

- Trunk/limb ratios
- Body surface area
- Blood pressure
- Heart rate
- Respiratory rate
- Fluid requirements
- Peak expiratory flow rate values
- Nutritional requirements
- Drug dosage
- Maturation of renal function
- Drug distribution and metabolism
- Ability to communicate
- Ability to understand
- Varying rate of maturation and development.

PHYSIOLOGICAL FACTS: DID YOU KNOW THAT . . .

- The blood volume of a 3-kg newborn is a mere *250 ml* (Fig. 11.3).

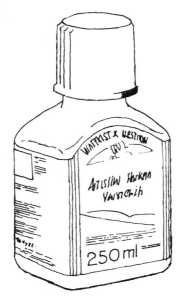

Fig. 11.3 3-kg newborn blood volume = 250 ml.

- In the first year of life, a baby increases in weight 3-fold and head circumference increases by one-third.
- The newborn liver is palpable because it is very active and a relatively very large organ.
- The 1-year-old's head circumference (and by inference brain size) at 47 cm is 85% of the average adult head at 55 cm.
- An average 2-year-old measuring 85 cm is *half* of completed adult height (Fig. 11.4).
- A palpable spleen is by implication about twice its normal size.
- A useful rule of thumb for normal peak expiratory flow rate (PEFR) in children is 30 × age in years + 30. A 6-year-old's PEFR is therefore about 210 l/min.
- Approximate systolic blood pressure in children = 100 + age in years ± 20 mmHg from age 5 years.

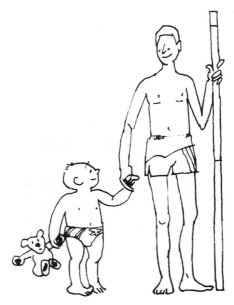

Fig. 11.4 Two-year-old = half adult height.

- Approximate diastolic blood pressure in children = 60 + age in years ± 15 mmHg from age 5 years.
- The average primary schoolchild aged 5–10 years should grow 5–7 cm each year.
- There is a 100-fold difference in weight between your smallest paediatric patients (600–800 g preterm) and your largest teenagers (60–80 kg and more). Think of the effect of this on drug dosages.

AT WHAT AGE CAN A CHILD . . .

Swallow a tablet?
Swallow a capsule?
Self-inject with insulin?

Do a finger prick blood glucose?
Competently perform peak flow rate?
Cooperate in a 24-hour urine collection?
Understand the concept of a clinical trial?
Consent to treatment?
Self-catheterize?
Hold inspiration for a chest radiograph?
Undergo MRI scan without sedation?
Cooperate for formal respiratory function testing (FEV, FVC, etc.)?

The answer, of course, is that there is no one correct answer. Children acquire skills at varying ages, mature at different stages, and achieve competencies more related to maturation than to chronological age (Fig. 11.5).

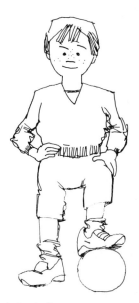

Fig. 11.5 Well boy with football.

SOME LATIN TRANSLATIONS

Erythema multiforme: redness of many shapes
Icterus: jaundice
Morbilliform: measles like
Pectus carinatum: pigeon chest
Pectus excavatum: funnel chest
Pediculosis capitis: head lice (nits)
Purpura fulminans: fulminant purpura
Status asthmaticus: severe progressive asthma
Status epilepticus: continuous epileptic seizure
Varicelliform: resembling chickenpox

A QUESTION OF FIVES

Most, but not all, of the answers are to be found in the text.
Give it a go:

- 5 causes of acute wheeze
- 5 Is associated with eczema
- 5 Ds for epiglottis
- 5 reasons for doing male circumcision
- 5 causes of macrocephaly (large head)
- 5 causes of microcephaly (small head)
- 5 types of hip disease in children
- 5 causes of meningism (stiff neck)
- 5 causes of bacterial meningitis
- 5 causes of acute stridor/croup
- 5 viruses causing red rash
- 5 features of Kawasaki's disease
- 5 Ss for assessing asthma
- 5 causes of bloody diarrhoea
- 5 causes of generalized lymphadenopathy
- 5 live vaccines
- 5 major features of rheumatic fever
- 5 components of the Apgar score
- 5 inborn errors of metabolism

- 5 bacteria causing UTIs
- 5 features of Henoch–Schönlein syndrome
- 5 injuries suggestive of child abuse
- 5 methods of collecting a urine sample
- 5 signs of dehydration
- 5 causes of hand tremor
- 5 types/causes of nappy rash
- 5 causes of abdominal distension
- 5 features of innocent/physiological murmur
- 5 signs of joint inflammation
- 5 serious lower respiratory pathogens

MULTIPLE CHOICE QUESTIONS (MCQS) – BEST OF FIVE

1. Blood pressure in the newborn infant is best measured by:
   A. Standard sphygmomanometry
   B. Automated machine
   C. Doppler ultrasonic
   D. Swan–Ganz catheter
   E. Palpatory method

2. The greatest health advance for children in the twentieth century was:
   A. Safe anaesthesia
   B. Newborn screening
   C. Antibiotics
   D. Immunization
   E. Oral rehydration

3. A 3-cm operative scar in the right lower quadrant is most likely to be:
   A. Laparoscopy
   B. Inguinal herniotomy
   C. Pyloromyotomy
   D. Orchidopexy
   E. Appendectomy

4. A 2-year-old child presents with tachypnoea 60/minute and grunting. The most likely diagnosis is:
   A. Laryngotracheobronchitis
   B. Bronchitis
   C. Acute asthma
   D. Pneumonia
   E. Foreign body

5. Which of the following causes of bacterial meningitis is most likely to result in 'brain damage':
   A. Meningococcal
   B. Pneumococcal
   C. *Haemophilus influenzae*
   D. *Listeria*
   E. Tubercular

6. The most likely explanation of acute inspiratory stridor in a 2-year-old child is:
   A. Epiglottis
   B. Foreign body
   C. Laryngotracheobronchitis
   D. Laryngomalacia
   E. Acute allergic laryngitis

7. An easily palpable enlarged spleen is at least:
   A. 2 times normal size
   B. 3 times normal size
   C. 4 times normal size
   D. 5 times normal size
   E. 6 times normal size

8. The most important component of the Apgar score is:
   A. Colour
   B. Muscle tone
   C. Reflex irritability
   D. Respiratory effort
   E. Heart rate

9. Of the conditions screened at birth by the 'heel-prick test' (Guthrie), the most common in Caucasians is:
   A. Phenylketonuria
   B. Cystic fibrosis
   C. Congential hypothyroidism
   D. Galactosaemia
   E. Haemochromatosis

10. The most common explanation of abdominal distension in Caucasian children is:
   A. Constipation
   B. Fluid
   C. Flatus
   D. Fat
   E. Organomegaly

11. The best clinical sign of intravascular volume depletion is:
   A. Reduces skin turgor
   B. Cold feet
   C. Slow capillary refill
   D. Sunken eyes
   E. Impalpable dorsalis pedis pulse

12. An 18-month-old boy, weighing 20 kg, is not walking. The most probable explanation is:
   A. Muscular dystrophy
   B. Developmental delay
   C. Dislocated hips
   D. Overweight
   E. Hypotonic

13. Drug dose in children is usually related to:
   A. Weight
   B. Renal function
   C. Body surface area
   D. Age
   E. Blood volume

14. The commonest explanation for a large head (circumference 56 cm) in a 4-year-old child is:
    A. Hydrocephalus
    B. Space-occupying lesion
    C. Neurofibromatosis
    D. Bone disorder
    E. Familial macrocephaly

15. The blood volume of a well and healthy 5-kg infant is approximately:
    A. 1500 ml
    B. 500 ml
    C. 400 ml
    D. 1000 ml
    E. 750 ml

16. A 2-year-old child with acute hip pain and limp is most likely to have:
    A. Septic arthritis
    B. A slipped upper femoral epiphysis
    C. Transient synovitis of the hip
    D. A lower limb fracture
    E. Henoch–Schönlein syndrome

17. Anaphylactoid purpura (Henoch–Schönlein syndrome) cannot be diagnosed without:
    A. Joint swelling
    B. Purpura
    C. Abdominal pain
    D. Haematuria
    E. Proteinuria

18. The cardinal early symptom/sign of pyloric stenosis in a 6-week-old infant is:
    A. Constipation
    B. Abdominal distension
    C. Projectile vomiting
    D. Poor feeding
    E. Palpable pyloric tumour

19. The most appropriate normal systolic blood pressure for a quiet 1-year-old infant is:
    A. 60–70 mmHg
    B. 70–80 mmHg
    C. 80–90 mmHg
    D. 90–100 mmHg
    E. 110–120 mmHg

20. At 6 weeks of age, the most important achieved developmental milestone is:
    A. Loss of Moro response (reflex)
    B. Grasp response
    C. Head control
    D. Responsive smiling
    E. Rolling over

Answers

1. C	11. C
2. D	12. D
3. E	13. A
4. D	14. E
5. B	15. C
6. C	16. C
7. A	17. B
8. E	18. C
9. B	19. C
10. D	20. D

MULTIPLE CHOICE QUESTIONS (MCQS) – TRUE/FALSE

Multiple answers: Choose <u>all</u> the options that are correct/true for the statements below. You can choose more than one option.

1. An innocent/ functional/ physiological murmur:
   A. May have a diastolic component
   B. Varies with position
   C. Is heard between the scapulae
   D. May produce a vibratory thrill
   E. Is accentuated by fever/pyrexia

2. The following are rarely heard in children:
   A. Pleural rub
   B. Systolic ejection click
   C. Venous hum
   D. Renal artery bruit
   E. Atrial fibrillation

3. Signs of developmental dysplasia of the hip include:
   A. Limb shortening on affected side
   B. Delayed walking
   C. Reduced abduction of the affected hip
   D. Hip pain
   E. An audible 'clunk'

4. Bronchial breathing:
   A. Is normal in infants under 1 year
   B. Is heard in pneumonia
   C. Is a feature of bronchiolitis
   D. Never occurs in asthma
   E. Indicates lobar consolidation

5. Which of the following are normal in infants under 1 year of age?
   A. Upgoing plantar response
   B. Cremasteric reflex
   C. Blue sclera
   D. Unilateral Moro response
   E. Periodic respiration

6. Which of the following are suggestive of inflicted injury (child abuse)?
   A. Buttock bruises
   B. Skin bruises
   C. Ear petechiae/ bruises
   D. Forehead bruises
   E. Perinatal bruises

7. Urine can be coloured:
   A. White
   B. Pink
   C. Orange
   D. Black
   E. 'Coke' like

8. Children (between 1 and 2 years of age), generally, do not like:
   A. Strangers
   B. Having head circumference measured
   C. Having blood pressure measured
   D. Pulse oximetry
   E. Sweets

9. Rickets is manifested clinically by:
   A. Pallor
   B. Pedal oedema
   C. Expanded costochondral junctions
   D. Genu valgus
   E. Delayed closure of anterior fontanelle

10. Cyanosis gives clinical information on:
    A. Haemoglobin concentration
    B. Blood volume status
    C. Peripheral perfusion
    D. Oxygen saturation
    E. Cardiac function

11. An average child has achieved almost 50% of final height by age 2 years. This growth is driven by:
    A. Thyroxine
    B. Growth hormone
    C. Insulin-like growth factor 1 (IGF-1)
    D. Nutrition
    E. All of the above

12. Methods of locomotion in a 15-month-old infant include:
    A. Crawling
    B. Rolling
    C. Bear walking
    D. Bottom shuffling
    E. Hopping

13. The physiological factors which make infants prone to dehydration include:
    A. Breast feeding
    B. Large body surface area
    C. High fluid requirements
    D. Overheating at night
    E. Inability to concentrate urine

14. A stiff neck (meningism) is a recognized feature of:
    A. Torticollis
    B. Meningitis
    C. Dental abscess
    D. Upper lobe pneumonia
    E. Retropharyngeal abscess

15. An enlarged testis can be found in:
    A. Testicular torsion
    B. Leukaemia
    C. Klinefelter's syndrome (XXY)
    D. Mumps orchitis
    E. Fragile X syndrome

16. Causes of cleft lip/palate include:
    A. Anticonvulsants
    B. Trisomic syndromes
    C. Smoking in pregnancy
    D. Paternal age
    E. Familial disposition

17. Signs of acute lobar pneumonia caused by streptococcal
    pneumonia include:
    A. Pleural rub
    B. Dullness to percussion
    C. Herpes labialis (cold sore)
    D. Rusty sputum
    E. Wheeze

18. Desquamating rash is a feature of:
    A. Eczema
    B. Erysipelas
    C. Scarlet fever
    D. Kawasaki's disease
    E. Rubella

19. Napkin area rashes include:
    A. Candidiasis
    B. Psoriasis
    C. Seborrhoeic dermatitis
    D. Cellulitis
    E. Ammoniacal dermatitis

20. Dietary obesity in childhood is accompanied by:
    A. Tall stature
    B. Hepatomegaly
    C. Slipper upper femoral epiphysis
    D. Narcolepsy
    E. Raised systolic blood pressure

Answers

1. B, E	11. D
2. A, D, E	12. A, B, C, D
3. C	13. B, C
4. B, E	14. B, D, E
5. A, B, C	15. A, B, D, E
6. A, C, E	16. A, B, E
7. A, B, C, D, E	17. A, B, C, D
8. A, B, C	18. C, D
9. C, E	19. A, C, E
10. D	20. A, C, E

Index

Note: Page numbers in italics refer to images.